One Bodymind Series • Book 1

Seek Wisdom

The Modern Quest for Health and Sustainability

Keith Berndtson, MD

ISBN
978-1935867005
ISBN-10:
1935867008
Library of Congress Control Number:
2011929441

One Bodymind Press

One Bodymind, Ltd.
Park Ridge, Illinois

Contents

Seek Wisdom

Information is not knowledge.
Knowledge is not wisdom. Wisdom is not truth.

—Anonymous

Say you have persistent symptoms of pain and fatigue that puzzle your family doctor. A referral starts the conveyor belt. Your trail leads you from one doctor to the next. At each stop you undergo diagnostic procedures that shed little light on your symptoms. You finally receive a diagnosis by default because, apparently, every other possibility has been excluded. Your diagnosis feels more like a label that elucidates nothing convincing about what is causing your symptoms, or how best to treat them.

You feel like your doctors are guessing. You try the drugs they recommend but they don't work for you. Some make you feel worse. Months go by. You experience creeping irritation about the fact that not once have any of your doctors dug deep into the narrative of your illness in an attempt to understand why it unfolded the way it did. You believe that a deeper grasp of your story could inform a more effective approach to treatment.

In a fit of fancy, you decide to see a physician who specializes in a field that doesn't yet officially exist. You've heard it called *integrative medicine*, *functional medicine*, *holistic medicine*, and less professional sounding names, too. All you know is that the doctor took your history starting from the last time you felt perfectly well, and constructed a narrative rich with clues from which emerged, for the first time, some power to explain what you would need to do to get well. You followed the advice. It worked.

What happened? Ask the conventional doctor and you're likely to be told that it was just a placebo effect. Ask the doctor who helped you and you'll learn that you got well with the help of a *clinical systems biology* approach to chronic illness. This book explores the implications of this method for solving the complex health problems of living systems, from the ecosystems of the planet to the living system that is you.

Clinical systems biology combines methodical health narrative construction with an integrative assessment of the functional integrity of systems as a whole. You wouldn't think such an approach would be so hard to find in the medical mainstream, but it is. Here's why:

- Primary care physicians generally can't afford the time required to thoroughly scrub your narrative for clues as to whether your bodily systems are performing well as a team, and if not, why not.

- Medical specialists rarely venture beyond their narrow scope of interest; they leave integrative assessment to primary care.

Health plans reward this dysfunctional design using the money that they collect from you and your employer. The systems biology approach that the functional medicine doctor took to solve your health problems? That's not medicine. But that's how it is when patients and freethinking physicians have no control over how health plans define medical necessity. Your "plan"—the plan paid for with dollars earned by you—coerces physicians into doing what makes the most sense to the plan and its business and medical executives. A conveyor belt of patients handled by doctors under contract makes sense to them. *That's* medicine.

Clinical systems biology is the primary focus of a functional medicine approach to the care and prevention of chronic illness—an approach that makes a great deal of sense to the patients and physicians who use it. Functional medicine is a still-sprouting medical specialty; it lacks the clout needed to join the club of officially Board-certified medical specialties. That's a big reason why health insurers get away with paying it no mind. It's a pity because around the world functional medicine is bailing many thousands of patients out of health trouble where usual and customary medical care has failed to be of help.

The "clinical" part of clinical systems biology refers to the mind-set the clinician uses to help solve health-related problems. The "systems biology" part refers to a new imperative that applies to all forms of clinical problem solving: the need to investigate functional relationships at multiple levels within the systems of the whole. This imperative applies whether the subject in need of clinical help is the patient in the room, a species in its habitat, or a country suffering from a weak economy and a broken system of governance.

The clinical systems biology skills of the functional medicine physician are becoming the central feature of academic integrative medicine programs and community-based integrative medicine practices. Integrative medicine programs can offer a jumble of complementary and alternative medical services. Functional medicine anchors diverse integrative medicine services to reasonably scientific standards for patient-centered chronic illness prevention and care.

Despite the growing consumer demand for integrative clinical problem solving, most integrative medicine programs operate outside the medical mainstream, with quality standards that vary. Yet by performing unhurried evaluations that subject the patient's problems to both the zoom lens of the specialist and the wide-angle lens of the systems biologist, integrative physicians supply what many long-suffering patients were unable to find in their encounters with medical specialists or primary care doctors—a path to wellness.

Roughly sixty percent of medical school affiliated academic medical centers have yet to sponsor an integrative medicine program. This reluctant embrace of integrative medicine by the medical mainstream is understandable when you consider the relatively low revenues generated by such programs, and the medical center staff politics of letting a loosely credentialed specialty into a medical center ecosystem where it will compete with other specialties for income.

This may change as medical centers move toward income based on savings generated by lowering their costs of care. A clinical systems biology approach to chronic illness would provide a competitive lower cost option than ongoing mainstream evaluation of patients whose chronic illnesses remained unexplained despite prior thorough evaluations. The mainstream's lukewarm reception of integrative medicine in general, and of functional medicine in particular, reflects the deeper cause of what's wrong with our health system: the money's not in helping you stay well; it's in treating you once you're ill and prone to health crises.

The same could be said about our political and economic systems: the money and power are not in the health and sustainability of our society—they're in whatever makes money or otherwise creates and preserves the kind of influence that keeps public and personal accountability worries to a comfortable minimum.

There are signs that lack of accountability within our health care sector is about to change. By 2015, the Affordable Care Act hopes to have a system in place that pays physicians based on value, not volume. Health insurers are now experimenting with ways to pay health care providers for the clinical and cost results they produce rather than the claims they submit. The ongoing tussle will be about which parties get to define how results should be measured and rewarded or punished.

The Affordable Care Act is giving health insurers far more leverage within the sector, though insurers were the most vocal opponents of the Act. This will result in more costs being shifted onto consumers, employers, hospitals, and physicians. We are entering a new age of health care cost reduction in which the health insurance industry has the power to impose draconian changes on parties that have little power to negotiate the resulting rates of decline in their cash flow.

What health insurers do with their newfound leverage could be viewed as acts of courage, but it remains to be seen whether they will be the wise stewards of health care funds that they claim to be. The policy challenge is to reform the health care sector in a fair and orderly way as opposed to letting insurance crusaders pillage it.

What has gone missing through several decades of attempted American health care reform is genuine leverage for health care consumers. In policymaking circles a type of condescension prevails, which holds that consumers should not be allowed to alter the mechanics of the health care sector because the complexity of the machine is way over their heads. Better to let health plans and their allies decide what to do with the consumer's health care dollars.

The closest we have come to consumer-driven health care in this country was a deliberate move in the late 1990's toward health savings accounts and higher deductible insurance plans. These policy instruments are best suited to people who are well and have no need for healthcare; they do little to help the chronically ill save money or spend more wisely. In today's weak economy, deductibles and savings account balances are seen as discretionary income to be spent only in an emergency—hardly a form of buying power. Reticence to incur deductibles and co-pays keeps plan subscribers out of the doctor's office and results in elective surgeries being put off. Health insurers wind up paying out less for claims on the heels of getting their annual rate hikes approved. It is no surprise that the nation's largest health plans reported record profits in 2011.

The Affordable Care Act is forcing industry stakeholders to repair what's wrong with the financial mechanics of the heath care industry at the expense of what's wrong with the industry's mechanics of healing. Consumers are not invited into the discussion about upcoming changes because they are not real stakeholders; they are end-users with so little leverage that they can continue to be ignored by industry powers that be.

If consumers had a real stake with leverage, they would support a functional medicine approach to chronic illness care. They want more than medical specialists providing care with a narrow focus. They see primary care doctors providing a broader focus but in such hurried fashion as not to matter. What they struggle to access are physicians willing to take the time needed to construct a detailed health narrative and develop an integrative care plan that can address complex health problems from a whole person perspective.

Today's health care consumers are growing more sophisticated and well organized. They want a health care system that is adept at promoting optimal wellness. For today's smart health consumer, the time has come to either fix the broken relationship between primary care and specialty medicine, or abandon the system for a more patient-friendly model.

Chronic disease steals your dignity and drains your assets while shoving you toward disability and premature death, creating complicated burdens for your loved ones that may linger for years after you're gone. The best way to avoid costly skirmishes with chronic illness is to know what you're doing when it comes to caring for your own health. Since our health care sector is engineered to make money by treating disease, to become wise in the ways of self-care, there is a need for high quality sources of health wisdom and wellness support.

Wisdom may not be truth, but it creates more value than knowledge alone. Wisdom combines factual knowledge with values-driven judgments based on experience about what works. A higher form of collective wisdom is needed to get our health system on a course that can help us achieve our full wellness potential as individuals, and as a species. Our race of beings has come to dominate the only known home for life in the universe. We must become wiser in the ways of health and wellness.

Our treatment of the environment plays an important role in the global burden of chronic disease. The pollutants that accumulate in our bodies are also concentrating in the ecosystems of the world, causing problems that could last for many generations. If our species is to safeguard the health of the environment upon which it depends, we will have to learn what we're doing when it comes to caring for the living systems of the world.

Humanity's to-do list ought to sober us up. Raise the standard of living for the hungry and the poor? Check. Reverse the trends that now threaten the viability of living systems? Check. Keep weapons of mass destruction out of the hands of terrorists and lunatics? Check. Avoid overcooking the planet? Check. The list is long and we're falling behind. We'll eventually be forced to call upon the wisdom of the crowd to see if many clicks make little work. Why wait? Let's start now. Let's test the hypothesis that an enlightened and empowered network of conscientious citizen-consumers can drive healthy cultural change. The stage is set and waiting for us to begin the modern quest for health and sustainability.

The problems that beset us are so ingrained as to be hidden behind the things we attend to just to get through the day. The biggest threats to health and sustainability live unseen deep within the connective tissues of our cultural institutions. Achieving a state of national or global wellness seems unlikely without substantial corporate and institutional transparency and public accountability.

Politics and business as usual seem only capable of making our problems worse. Financial markets keep inviting new forms of unrestrained risk- and profit-taking. Industrial markets perpetuate pollution of our ecosystems and loot the world's natural resources. Consumers spend money that they don't have. Education fails to prepare young people for becoming knowledge workers in the new economy. Health care cost inflation steers us toward social and economic collapse. We fight terrorism, trying to make the world safe for democracy at a tremendous cost in blood and treasure, yet our insecurities mount with each passing year. Everywhere we look culture wars are being waged by enraged ideologues and their puppet masters, health and wellness be damned.

Where is the wisdom of the market? Where is the wisdom of good governance? Where is the wisdom of the public? Where is the wisdom of statecraft? Where is the wisdom of faith and reason working together? Where is the wisdom of human culture?

How is it that America's major institutions, which took shape as reflections of our histories, values, beliefs, and moral commitments, are losing their ability to secure the functional integrity of a society with such a proud history? What can be done to restore these institutions to their original purpose and effectiveness? What will it require of us as individuals to be healthy and happy in ways that encourage the health of the whole?

In this, the first book in the One Bodymind Series, I introduce the clinical systems biology approach to complex problem solving, and I explore how these concepts apply to personal wellness, cultural change, and social cooperation.

I begin with a look at integrative medicine and how its mindset can be used to improve the care of patients who either have chronic illness or are looking to delay its onset. I also look at what makes the culture of integrative medicine appealing to a growing number of physicians and health consumers.

Equipped with a clinical systems biology perspective, I call out the threat our species poses to biodiversity and environmental health. I then take an evolutionary look at why humanity bears a moral responsibility to become a better steward of the living systems of the earth, and why the concept of functional integrity should matter not just to science and medicine but also to religion and modern culture.

I look at the phenomenon of social evolution and how its progression of major transformations has implications for modern human adaptation within the Earth system. I consider our health and sustainability dilemma from a range of cultural viewpoints, and suggest how sources of wisdom should go about earning our trust.

From there I examine the supposed conflicts between faith and reason. The tensions between science and religion, objective and subjective experience, physics and metaphysics, random evolution and narrative heading in a direction—all seem to dissolve when viewed from within an integrative clinical mind-set.

The trail then turns within, to the inner world of human nature where variations on happiness and discontentment fight for our attention and the right to control how we experience life in the moment. In the context of how human values, ideals, and beliefs take shape, I indicate how science, religion, culture, and philosophy might best position themselves as a team to win our affections and promote health and sustainability.

I use thought experiment to discern answers to the question, "What would a doctor of planetary medicine advise humanity to do?" The answers, though insufficient, point us in the direction that evolution might head if it were converging on solutions to health and sustainability within systems as a whole.

The book concludes with our realization that we are players in the world's most epic game. If we underestimate our gifts, we undermine the potential of our species to become a healing force in the world—a force able to secure greater human flourishing for generations to come.

The primary purpose of this book is to ground the modern quest for health and sustainability in a clinical philosophy that can be used to tackle the most complex health problems facing people, the human species, and the vast, entangled web of living systems. The philosophical framework for the quest is clinical because it has a mission to heal systems whose dysfunction stands in the way of health and sustainability.

The quest is best equipped if it uses an integrative clinical mind-set to solve problems because it will not settle for diagnosis—it seeks to explain as fully as possible the causes of illness and dysfunction. The clinical philosophy of the quest is a form of *idealistic realism* whose practical consequence is to match our ideals—and the plans we base on them—to the requirements of biological reality. Anything less could undermine a quest whose purpose is to promote the health and sustainability of biological systems.

The 21st Century should witness science, government, business, religion, and culture forming new functional units capable of supporting health and sustainability across regions. In this process, the noble tradition of medicine must no longer be held hostage by third parties; the medical profession must regain the public trust and lead the quest whose aim is to make our species healthy and whole.

Perhaps we will someday see ourselves with righteous pride for how we came to support functional integrity within our spheres of influence, for how our cultures came to accept their roles as the world's own physician—stewards of health and sustainability within the greater whole, a proudly functioning part of the one bodymind that spans the cosmos.

Bodymind. The word bounces lightly off the tongue yet sounds foreign and unnecessary. It's not a part of common speech. You won't find it in urban dictionaries or the scientific lexicon. To convey the idea that being human has both physical and mental aspects that are hard to separate, the more familiar terms "body and mind" and "mind-body" seem suitable enough. Why use the word "bodymind"?

In the terms "body and mind" and "mind-body," the conjunction and the hyphen reinforce an artificial separation of body and mind that has held sway in medical thinking for far too long. Your body and mind are part of one whole. If it is unwise to separate them when attempting to solve complex clinical problems, it is unwise to separate them when attempting linguistic clarity. The word "bodymind" is far closer to the truth: it captures the fusion between energy and substance that characterizes the highly evolved living system that is you.

Laypeople looking for medical explanations quickly lose their way in thickets of jargon. Even professionals can have a hard time bushwhacking through the medical literature. All are challenged to decide where to find the best sources of health information. Are the sources unbiased? Did the right to edit content for this webpage go to the highest bidder? How should we sort sound science from savvy marketing? These challenges make it all the more important for health-minded consumers to be scrupulous about websites that aggregate health information.

Embattled consumers need a trustworthy guide in their search for wisdom on self-care and making best use of one's health care dollars. They will find such resources at *onebodymind.com*, where members and subscribers are building a wellness support plan that aims to create paths to health and wellness everywhere within its sphere of influence.

The time is ripe for a website that filters scientific knowledge, cultural traditions, and personal experience for their practical relevance to health and sustainability. Scientific knowledge alone will not save us. That said, scientific research has entered a period of grand inflation. Global output of scientific articles easily exceeds over half a million per year. If you read scientific articles at rate of two per day, like I try to do, you're already seven centuries behind.

According to the Royal Society's review of growth and change in global science, *Knowledge, Networks, and Nations: Global Scientific Collaboration in the 21st Century*, in 2011 seven million researchers around the world were collectively supported by funding topping $1 trillion, up forty-five percent compared to 2002. The fastest growth in scientific productivity is being seen in China, India, Brazil, and the Middle East. The United States, Europe, and Japan still account for the majority of funded research, language translation, and journal citations, but their numbers are decreasing relative to those in the countries with more rapidly expanding research enterprises.

Science is a vibrant, collaborative, multi-polar player in the globalization process. Scientists are better networked than ever before, and their cultural openness allows for vigorous integration of ideas and findings. If this were true for other institutions of human culture, we'd be evolving toward healthy and sustainable ways of being at something faster than a snail's pace. But alas, our best wisdom judges that scientific knowledge alone will never be enough to save us from ourselves.

With each passing month our scientific understanding of human biology reinforces the notion that our bodyminds are pro-grammed to win; remove the obstacles, and it is fair to assume that your bodily systems will automatically resume working to heal and sustain their functional integrity as a team. Yet the med-ical literature describes little of what could be described as the wisdom of the human bodymind, let alone what can be done, medically speaking, to tap into what could well be described as the most powerful medicine in the world.

The social network taking shape at *onebodymind.com* will sup-port the introduction of new perspectives into scientific discus-sions about bodymind wisdom, and about summoning the wis-dom needed to confront our major global challenges. The Royal Society acknowledges the need for a better integration of ideas at the social level. The paper's authors write:

> Global challenges are interdependent and interrelated: climate change, water, food and energy security, popu-lation change, and loss of biodiversity are all intercon-nected. The dynamic between these issues is complex, yet many global assessment and research programs are

managed separately, often reflecting lack of coordination in the policy sphere.

The need for better research coordination spurs innovation. Demonstration projects are underway. But we need a wisdom-seeking process for interpreting, discussing, and making practical sense of the rising tide of scientific research findings. The authors anticipate a gradual learning process:

> Global challenges are being addressed via a number of different organizational mechanisms: through intergovernmental or international bodies, through national systems, and by private individuals and corporations. These mechanisms often deploy novel and innovative forms of partnership, some of which work well, others less so.

The Royal Society then makes a point that could serve as the main thesis of this book:

> Science is essential for addressing global challenges, but it cannot do so in isolation. A wide range of approaches will be required, including the appropriate use of financial incentives, incorporating non-traditional forms of knowledge, and working with the social sciences and wider disciplines. Science is crucial but it is unlikely to produce all the answers by itself: the science infrastructure works best when it is supported by, and enables, other systems.

It is encouraging that the international scientific community is forming new channels for data sharing and communication, and new ways of partnering to usher in new solutions to difficult problems. Yet it cannot realize its full problem solving potential without insight from the social sciences and from culturally determined ways of learning and managing knowledge.

Most scientific papers focus on narrow slivers of subject matter. If science is to influence cultural change it will need to contextualize its findings and address the practical concerns of varied cultural audiences. The biggest challenge for the scientific community is to translate its conclusions into practical applications that win the favor of public and private institutions not just for their narrow benefits but also for the social meaning and health relevance of its findings.

The scientific community needs to do a better job of filtering out the junk data, selective reporting, and marketing bias that contaminate much of the world's published research, and do so knowing that private sources of funding may not be pleased with the results. As with clinical medicine, where subjective elements of decision-making are needed to meet the health challenges of the chronically ill, subjective elements of decision-making are needed to fulfill the quest for global health and sustainability. The value of non-traditional knowledge is its ability to contribute to reliably positive outcomes without total clarity regarding the detailed causative mechanisms at work. Intuition, personal experience, and the wisdom of the crowd all have a role to play in solving the complex problems of living systems.

In addition to a clinical, wisdom-based orientation toward its task, the quest for health and sustainability will also fare better with a balanced interaction between centralizing and decentralizing forces, as this helps to balance against the asymmetrical advantages that tend to accrue to established, centralized sources of power.

In *The Starfish and the Spider*, authors Ori Brafman and Rod Beckstrom contrast the difference between centralized and decentralized organizations:

A centralized organization is easy to understand. You have a clear leader who's in charge, and there's a specific place where decisions are made. This organizational type is coercive because the leaders call the shots: when a CEO fires you, you're out.

In a decentralized organization, there's no clear leader, no hierarchy, and no headquarters. If and when a leader does emerge, that person has little power over others. The best that person can do to influence people is to lead by example...This [is] an open system, because everyone is entitled to make his or her own decisions.

Brafman and Beckstrom clarify:

A coercive system is not necessarily bad. Rules need to be set and enforced or the system collapses. But when a coercive system takes on an open system whose activities are unwelcome, the decentralized organization tends to become even more open and decentralized.

When the music labels first took on Napster, the hub that allowed users to share music files for free, they learned that the organization was more like a starfish than a spider. A centralized organization is like a spider, in that you can squash its head and your problem is gone. Napster was decentralized. The entity had no rules or internal enforcers that the music industry's legal eagles could control with lawsuits. They eventually won a Supreme Court decision against Napster, but new free rider music file-sharing services sprang up. Cut the leg off a starfish, and it'll grow a new one because its metabolic systems are highly decentralized.

Wisdom grows one brushstroke at a time. Most centralized organizations are coercive systems that use large brushes to paint a picture that favorably depicts their corporate interests. A decentralized network of conscientious citizen-consumers has the potential to leverage that kind of corporate behavior and paint a more sustainable scenario by using millions of tiny brushes at a time. Humanity's current big picture is mainly composed of large brushstrokes that reveal an unsustainable system of cultures. A decentralized, non-coercive effort to mobilize millions of little brushes might change the picture into a scene with a more hopeful future.

The big picture is always changing and thus unfinished, but over time we need it to encourage us to believe that we are growing more capable of creating a healthier, more sustainable path into the future; that together we can agree on how to move from what is to what ought to be.

This book addresses an unusual question: What would a wise planetary medicine doctor advise humanity to do to improve its prospects for long-term health and sustainability? I approach the task of answering this as a clinician who is curious to learn whether some collaborative mix of logical analysis and subjective experience might yield an answer that feels compelling and agreeable across a range of cultural perspectives.

Since it is not possible to draw the line between where a body ends and a mind begins—or where a mind ends and a culture begins—it is fair to say that no bodymind stands alone. Each one of us is a complex whole made up of many lesser parts, and together we are but a part of an astoundingly greater whole.

Our toughest problems are clinical in the sense that they are too complex for simple, rules-based solutions. As much as health plans try to distill medical practice down to some sort of rules-based essence, their policies are no match for the true complexity of chronic health problems. A different, more functional vision of health and healing is required. From the patient with chronic pain and fatigue to the species looking to protect its environment while raising the standard of living for billions of people, problems this complex will not submit to algorithmic solutions. Surely they will not be solved using narrow mind-sets or inflexible ideologies.

As you reflect upon the failure of current ideologies to solve our health and sustainability dilemmas, turn your mind to the ancient path that our ancestors took to get us where we are today. Is global social transformation possible? Can we shift the story from a game of thrones to a game of health and sustainability? Can we find the path that leads to a more dignified global standard of living *and* responsible stewardship of the natural world that sustains us? Our modern quest is to locate such a path and follow it as far as we possibly can.

As you move through the books of the One Bodymind Series, imagine yourself moving along this path. You will meet the minds of many thinkers whose ideas relate in some unforeseen way to health and sustainability. You may begin to see some "already decided" things in a new way. Some of your deeply held values and beliefs may evolve to accommodate new ways of thinking. In the way a river joins the ocean, or a germ in a seed grows, the edifices of cultural intolerance may give way to a higher functional imperative—one that mandates the creation of a multicultural infrastructure for the wisdom of wellness.

We live in an age where social media has become a promising new tool for solving complex clinical problems. If crowd-accelerated innovation is needed anywhere, it is in securing the functional integrity of institutions and industry sectors whose broken ways are becoming the leading source of chronic illness within the larger web of ecosystems. The capacity to spread ideas amounts to little unless we have ideas worth spreading. To effectively promote health and sustainability, we'll have to acknowledge what they require of us.

Before setting out on this expedition, we must prepare to contest with ideas from cultural realms whose worldviews conflict. Our mission, in a sense, is to pull ideas from science, religion, philosophy, culture, politics, and business in search of a consensus on what long-standing health and sustainability will require of our species.

To make our way along the perilous path of competing worldviews, we'll want the advantages and benefits of a full clinical mind-set.

The Power of a
Full Clinical Mind-set

◇◇◇◇◇◇◇◇◇◇◇◇◇◇◇◇◇◇◇◇◇◇◇◇◇◇◇◇◇◇◇◇

In medicine we contend with complex systems for a living. We bring to our task a generic problem-solving template, or clinical mind-set, which operates as follows:

1. Assess what's going on.

2. Make a diagnosis.

3. Set treatment goals.

4. Treat to fit the diagnosis and reach treatment goals.

5. Monitor what happens.

6. Reassess what's going on, in light of what's been happening.

7. Adjust as needed to keep moving closer to treatment goals.

With this problem-solving mind-set, the results you get depend most heavily on the strength of your assessments. If the thought-product of steps one or six are weak, your results will also be weak.

You might assume that for chronic illness the best clinical problem solving occurs when doctors and insurers design and implement evidence-based disease management programs. This is incorrect.

The best problem solving for chronic health problems occurs when clinicians use an integrative clinical mind-set centered on the unique functional needs of each patient. The results, as with any problem solving mind-set, depend on the quality of the assessment. Integrative clinical thinkers assess chronic health problems by building a detailed narrative of the patient's illness history. They do so looking for ways to explain why loss of function unfolded as it did so treatment can take aim at the roots of the patient's problems.

To make ends meet, many primary care physicians are forced by insurance reimbursement rules to take short cuts when assessing complex health problems—a form of coercion that works against the better clinical judgment of caring physicians who want the information that a detailed illness narrative can provide, but who must settle for less for reasons of getting paid by those who make the rules. The difference between an integrative, narrative-based assessment and a third party payment-driven abridged assessment is akin to the difference between a Frontline documentary and sound bite.

This observation is based on evidence found less in medical journals and more from patients who have experienced the benefits of an integrative clinical approach to care, where in many cases conventional, evidence-based medicine guidelines have already had their turn and failed to produce the results sought by the patient.

Jeffery Bland, PhD, a co-founder of the Institute for Functional Medicine, has long championed the view that health is a dynamic balance of multiple systems whose web-like interactions must be taken into account if patients are to maintain healthy organ reserves and experience vitality past an average life span. Bland teaches and conducts research in the field of nutrigenomics. In his 1999 book, *Genetic Nutritioneering*, Bland wrote, "Our genes are in constant communication with the foods that we eat, and they are taking their orders from the nutrients and phytochemicals in our diet." Research since then amply demonstrates the truth of this observation.

Vitamins, minerals, and plant-derived micronutrients (phyto-nutrients) are woven into our physiology. They have long been in conversation with the evolving human bodymind, whereas drugs, most of which are new to nature, have only recently opened their conversation with us.

Systems biology science reveals how phytonutrients help nudge dysfunctional cellular systems back into balance. This is something our ancestors came to understand based upon careful clinical observation. Doctors who recognize the importance of plant-based nutrition know it through the ancient art of clinical observation as well, but we also have the advantage of knowing it through research advances involving cell signaling, regulation, and metabolism.

Dr. Bland's team at the Functional Medicine Research Center in Gig Harbor, Washington, has shown that plant extract combinations can alter cell-signaling pathways by dialing down the over-expression of inflammation-promoting genes. No anti-inflammatory drug on the market or in development has even the theoretical ability to reach so deeply and elegantly into the biology of your cells.

Dr. Bland's *Future of the Clinic* seminar used a Youtube video to drive home the point that our medical-industrial complex is missing the criticality of nutrition and lifestyle change as a metabolic balancing force in cell biology. To take this test, go to Youtube, search "dothetest," and watch the video, or go to www.dothetest.co.uk/basketball.html.

By rough estimate, only 1 percent of the 950,000 doctors in the United States are equipped to practice functional medicine. Considering the entire physician fleet, the number of functional medicine doctors amounts to a rounding error. Like me, most of these doctors have picked up their functional medicine experience in bits and pieces during the course of their careers. High-quality certification programs in functional medicine have only recently gotten under way.

Most functional medicine physicians have strong conventional medical credentials. Many have additional skills in complementary and alternative medicine but not all integrative physicians possess similar levels of functional medicine skill.

In mainstream health care, specialty medicine is fragmented into various silos of expertise. If your health problem falls within the range of this expertise, the specialist's standard of care will typically help you achieve certain disease management goals. If the specialist does not have an answer, you are sent back to your primary care doctor, perhaps with a suggestion about arranging consultation with a different type of specialist.

The primary care physician inherits the rhetoric of whole-person care, but schedules are so packed that it becomes hard for the primary care doctor to get through his or her checklist in a fifteen-minute visit. Insurers coach patients to come to their doctor visit prepared with a full list of questions. The visit turns into a contest between a doctor who needs to run through a checklist while documenting everything a certain way or risk a denied claim, and the patient who wants answers to multiple questions and who hopes for a physician who will hear the full story behind the symptoms. In primary care the gap between rhetoric and practice is disturbingly wide.

Patients with chronic illness can get caught between specialty care that is deep but narrow and primary care that is broad but shallow and short on time. An integrative, clinical systems biology approach corrects this problem by encouraging the doctor to systematically construct a health narrative with depth and range. Clues to a patient's biological imbalances are seen more readily in the context of a carefully crafted narrative that sees the long arc of the story and can put a magnifier on the story's episodic slides into chronic illness. A thorough health narrative is especially useful in cases where chronic illness remains medically unexplained by, but non-responsive to, usual and customary care.

Mainstream medical problem solving focuses hard on fitting people into diagnostic categories, where each diagnosis points to a current set of best practices. These best practices have a tendency to look like an inventory of drugs and procedures ready to be deployed at each station along the conventional care conveyor belt. The importance of lifestyle change is acknowledged, but the support systems to promote healthy lifestyles are weak. No approach to chronic illness prevention or care can be considered a best practice without systematic attempts to place dietary and nutritional advice in the context of your unique history, biochemistry, and, when warranted, your genetics.

One of the common frustrations with the current mainstream approach to chronic illness is the tendency toward *polypharmacy*. This refers to the personal use of multiple prescription drugs and/ or over-the-counter drugs, often in doses or quantities greater than needed to obtain health benefits.

Medication lists have a habit of growing longer with time. Whenever a new symptom pops up, the doctor may prescribe another drug to swat it down. If that drug causes a side effect, well, to quote Stephen Colbert, chief spokesperson for Prescott Pharmaceuticals, "We have a medication for every ailment, including the ailments caused by our previous medications."

In *Detoxification and Healing*, Sidney MacDonald Baker, MD, notes, "There are only so many ways of *being* sick, but there are many ways of *getting* sick." He refers to functional medicine as an "alternative to mainstream medicine that focuses on balance within the individual as contrasted to treatment of disease."

The key differences in the clinical mind-set employed by practitioners using a clinical systems biology approach to chronic health problems:

1. Assess what's going on.

2. *Formulate a working explanation* for the person's illness.

3. Set treatment goals.

4. *Treat to restore functional integrity to the system as a whole.*

5. Monitor what happens.

6. Reassess what's going on, in light of what's been happening.

7. *Adjust as needed to keep restoring balanced function within the whole.*

Commenting on the mainstream chronic illness paradigm, Baker noted, "Once a doctor has made a diagnosis, thinking can stop and prescribing can start." Once the diagnosis is made, we act like "we know what you've got and here's what you should take for it" so we can move on to the next patient.

By contrast, in a functional medicine approach, diagnoses are much like labels—they orient us to your brand of illness, but the label itself doesn't explain what we want to know about how you got sick.

The search for explanations pulls doctor and patient deeper into the clinical story, to find clues about what led to what's going on now. It is a search that doesn't end unless and until goals are met and a system for building self-care skills has become part of the patient's routine. With a clinical systems biology approach, it takes a long time to reach the conclusion, "That's all we can do."

In a conventional medical setting, once a diagnosis is made, it often feels to the patient as if the search for explanations has come to an abrupt end. A cookbook treatment is chosen—combine 10 mg of this with 25 mg of that and simmer for six weeks—and thereafter what happens to your disease markers may seem more important than what happens to you.

Mainstream health institutions have taken little notice of functional medicine so far, although this is beginning to change. The mainstream seems far more enamored with another conceptual approach to improving the quality of health care that goes by the moniker, *evidence-based medicine.*

Evidence-based practice is defined as the integration of best research evidence with clinical expertise and patient values to guide medical decision-making. The practical goal of this movement is to reduce medical errors and practice variations. In the name of best research evidence, however, the evidence-based practice movement runs the risk of throwing out good practice variations along with the bad.

Evidence-based medicine has a bias toward the *randomized controlled trial*, or RCT. The RCT is a study design that minimizes bias by randomizing research subjects into experimental and control groups. When subjects have an equal chance of being assigned to receive an intervention (experimental subjects) or go without intervention (the controls), study results stand a better chance of determining cause-effect relationships. If functional medicine has little RCT evidence to go by, then it has little chance of measuring up. It doesn't seem to matter that functional medicine relies on the evidence of patient care outcomes caused by multidimensional interventions based on a solid grasp of the kind of foundational biological imbalances that yield power to explain a given patient's problems.

Studies that are not randomized and controlled do suffer from more types of bias, and are less reliable at identifying causes and effects. Despite this advantage, RCTs have many disadvantages. They are expensive, difficult to do well, and perhaps most troubling, their findings apply to strictly defined groups of research subjects, making it difficult for the doctor to translate RCT findings to the unique patient. RCTs are supposed to make life easier for the physician. RCTs are supposed to take the guesswork out of practicing medicine so physicians can move patients through at ever increasing speeds.

Evidence-based medicine has its fair share of success stories. Yet on the whole, evidence-based medicine speeds up the patient conveyor belt with the help of data that do not extrapolate well from the experimental group to the individual patient in need of care plans that are tailored to fit his or her unique situation.

The evidence-based medicine movement ignores the functional medicine precept that people get sick in different ways—that they can arrive at the same diagnosis by different routes—and that they should therefore be treated in a way that takes into account their unique history, biochemistry, and genetics.

When setting up experimental and control groups, the RCT design team attempts to equalize their differences, whereas the clinical systems biologist is trying to do just the opposite: clarify and factor in what makes each case different from the next.

There's nothing wrong with wanting to base medical practice on good scientific evidence, but good medical practice also requires the clinical skill to tackle health problems that reliable RCTs have yet to illuminate—and given their complexity, that amounts to almost all chronic health problems.

The risk to society is this: if the evidence-based medicine movement simply puts new clothing on the old concept of "name the disease, name the drug for the disease," doctors will enact a mechanized, force-fed approach to chronic illness that neglects the importance of biochemical individuality, therapeutic lifestyle change, and the strategic uses of plant-based nutrition—essential concepts for the clinical systems biologist that, due to the complexity that they introduce to physician's task, are not as amenable to study by means of RCTs.

Evidence-based medicine is a branch that grows from the more valuable root concept of *informational literacy*, which refers to a doctor's ability to recognize when additional information is needed, and to understand how to locate it, evaluate it, and effectively put it into play when that is the case. Functional medicine is a different, perhaps more robust branch that grows from the same root concept.

Keith Posley, MD, and colleagues at the Stanford University School of Medicine, teach an informational literacy approach. They encourage physicians and students to humbly and flexibly recognize when more information is needed to guide the patient. The most valuable information more often comes from the patient than the medical literature. This model is tailored more to the needs of the physician as learner and healer than to the needs of policy makers looking to forge the plowshares of research into swords raised against freethinking medical practice variations.

More is at stake here than the future of America's health system. Hanging in the balance is whether Americans will continue to reward a system bent toward managing disease rather than preventing disease and promoting wellness. This will depend on how seriously we take the task of learning what disease prevention and wellness promotion requires of us.

I am hopeful that once Americans understand more about health in the big picture, they will demand a more robust and flexible paradigm for evaluating evidence about what works to produce wellness. Once stirred, an empowered health consumer movement could summon the leverage to steer health sector markets toward more effective methods for creating, restoring, and maintaining wellness at personal and public levels.

Businesses in the heath care sector are hardwired to resist changes that would result in a loss of power and influence. They have an uncanny ability to manipulate legislation from the side-lines. They'd have less power to maneuver past the market prefer-ences of consumers—the individuals and employers who are pay-ing most of the bills—but consumers lack solidarity and stressed employers favor any policy, good or bad for health, that will lower their costs. A piece to the puzzle is to position consumers to pres-sure health sector institutions to stop oversimplifying the com-plexity of our chronic health problems.

Chronic illness is a complex puzzle for which third party-driven snap judgments are no match. The best practices in con-ventional medicine have a habit of turning to the same tools: conclusions from masterfully spun drug company-sponsored RCTs. These skillfully marketed studies routinely neglect the web-like complexity of systems biology reality; they miss what they're not looking for.

Based on a widely cited analysis done by John Ioannidis, MD, DSc, at least 30 percent of published RCT findings, and up to 80 percent of all published research findings, miss the truth.

We cannot sustain our costly habit of waiting until people become diagnosable with a disease, then treating the disease in a reflexive way that overvalues the statistical significance of sin-gle variable interventions while neglecting the nuances of what makes each case different on the whole. Banking on rescue drugs and procedures ignores what was happening in the run-up to the illness, where multidimensional assessment and less costly options could have prevented the illness or long delayed its onset. It also ignores the long evolutionary conversation between our cells and the nutrients that guide our genomes toward health or disease.

A functional medicine-driven systems biology approach to clinical problem solving moves beyond diagnoses toward deeper working explanations of—and lower cost solutions to—chronic health problems.

The wise health consumer will make it his or her business to ascertain at the front end of a health care encounter whether the problem-solving framework in play has the ability to handle the multiple layers of systems interaction that goes on in most chronic illnesses. Framed certificates are just office décor; they don't answer the question about whether the medical paradigm being used can effectively contend with the unique puzzle of your complex health problems. Good word of mouth is more dependable, but not always available.

To make life easier for health consumers, would-be solvers of chronic health problems should declare in advance what problem-solving framework they're using to power their clinical mind-sets. For health consumers and providers alike, there are three clinical mind-sets from which to choose:

Conventional medicine:

Nothing is valid until it is proven to be valid.

Alternative medicine:

Anything is valid until it is proven to be invalid.

Integrative medicine:

Whatever works.

I have traveled in all three worlds. It's not hard to find the good, the bad, and the ugly in each one, but in my experience wellness seekers are better served by an integrative clinical mind-set that can combine the strengths of the conventional and alternative mind-sets. The integrative mind-set has a thirst for evidence and a license to use experience and intuition when evidence falls short; it is a fully equipped mind-set.

I believe that our medical generalists would make great integrative doctors if they weren't stuck in practice settings that forced them to see too many patients in a day and be all things to all people. Medical specialists would also make great integrative doctors if they were willing and able to deviate from business as usual.

Integrative doctors have an unusually high tolerance for ambiguity—a trait frowned upon in emergency departments, intensive care units, and operating rooms where most medical decisions can and should be based on rules and algorithms. But the care and prevention of chronic illness is vastly more complex than we make it out to be. Because of its complexity, chronic illness is hard to manage using rules and algorithms alone. Tolerance for ambiguity affords the integrative doctor more flexibility when it comes to fitting a care plan to the needs of the patient as an individual. There are too few integrative thinkers in medicine. There are too few integrative thinkers, period.

I didn't start out thinking this way.

Slipping Out of the Mainstream

◇◇◇◇◇◇◇◇◇◇◇◇◇◇◇◇◇◇◇◇◇◇◇◇◇◇◇◇◇◇◇◇◇

Ten years into my practice as a family doctor I had a life-changing experience. I was an instructor at an academic medical center, where I ran the corporate health program. A top executive with a Fortune 100 company came to me for a physical. At the end of the visit, he asked me for advice on behalf of his sister, whose four-year-old daughter was scheduled to have tubes put through her eardrums to relieve pressure caused by frequent ear infections. His sister wasn't totally sold on the idea and wondered what I might advise. I told him that tubes are the way to go if the recurrent infections might endanger the child's hearing.

A year later he returned and led off the visit with, "Remember my niece with the ear problems?"

"Sure," I said, "how'd she do with surgery?"

"She didn't need it."

"What happened?"

"They took her to a holistic doctor. He took her off dairy and wheat, did a few other things, and you know what? It solved the problem."

"That's great!"

"Great?" he said, leaning his face closer to mine. "Our company and employees pay an arm and a leg for answers to problems like this. Are you telling me we have to leave the system and pay again so our kids can avoid surgery? Whose job is it to know the options?"

The words were like a bullet train roaring through my head.

He was being stern but friendly, like an operations chief who wants his team to run things as well as possible and then even better. Still, I couldn't help but feel embarrassed for myself and for my profession.

This was the last straw in a burden of similar patient encounters in which executives called me to task for not being knowledgeable enough about natural therapies for various problems. So I gave it serious thought when Dr. David Edelberg approached me with a job offer. David, a widely respected integrative physician then and now, informed me that his business plan was backed by venture capital and that the financing could guarantee my salary.

After some trepidation, I decided to leave my medical center position to join his holistic practice with the idea that I'd close some knowledge gaps about natural therapies, sort out what worked, and, if the stock option plan tanked, head back to academia with an integrative medicine program proposal.

As fate would have it, after four years spent building an advanced integrative medicine practice model in four regions of the country, the company shifted its focus and divested itself of all health care operating risk. This meant the doctors and practitioners had to make new practice arrangements. Though disappointed by the business outcome, I came away richer from having been mentored by an exemplary group of integrative clinicians during what for me amounted to a four-year fellowship in integrative medicine. I opted to keep cultivating my clinical systems biology skills, and co-founded a practice that would major in integrative medicine with a minor in primary care.

I came to learn that, if allowed, a rising tide of non-reimbursed primary care work swamps an integrative approach to care. Treading the water of primary care was forcing me to let go of my capacity to provide a deeper, more studied approach to chronic illness. I decided to close my practice to new primary care patients, believing that I could accomplish more good helping patients who were inexplicably unwell despite usual medical care.

I remained an independent, community-based doctor. Without a champion in the upper ranks, trying to establish an integrative foothold in an academic medical center can be an exercise in frustration if the prevailing culture frowns upon divergent thinking. So in 2007 I started over with a handpicked practice team, and we set out to develop a scalable clinical systems biology practice model.

My allegiance to clinical systems biology was forged early in my experience as an integrative medicine physician. During my first week as a fledgling holistic doctor, back in the summer of 1996, I had a case that changed the way I view the patient-doctor relationship. A pale woman with sunken eyes told me she hadn't slept well for seven months because Emma, her fifteen-month-old daughter, suffered from eczema so bad that she was scratching her cheeks raw and crying most of the night. She had recently taken Emma to see a dermatologist at the children's hospital down the street, who recommended a more potent steroid cream—the third increase in six months.

The woman was glad that the cream worked, but she didn't want to settle for treating symptoms alone. She knew the end game; regular use of potent steroid creams creates problems of its own. She had done her homework and was seeking alternative perspective to get at the root cause of her daughter's problem.

I confessed that I had been on the job for only two days and that I wasn't yet a natural medicine expert, but that I, too, wanted to know more about alternative options for health problems. "Perfect!" she said, "Your mind is open. You don't know how hard it is to find an open-minded doctor these days." She helped me feel content with the idea that our acting like graduate students trying to figure something out together was fine. It has felt fine to me ever since.

Emma's eczema appeared shortly after she started eating solid foods, so her mother wanted me to check for delayed food sensitivities, something I'd never done before. I went ahead and ordered a blood panel that an allergist colleague had told me was misleading because it measured a "normal" antibody response to food proteins.

The allergy research literature describes this type of antibody as having a protective, blocking function. In this case, blood levels might simply reflect what the body does naturally. My integrative colleagues agreed, but they insisted that certain patterns could reflect clinically significant abnormalities. They reasoned that if there were unusually high antibody levels in response to a few foods, or moderately elevated antibody levels to an unusually broad range of foods, that it raises the question, "Why is the immune system working *so hard* to block food proteins that it should be able to tolerate?"

The test showed that Emma was producing unusually high amounts of blocking antibody specific to eggs, dairy, wheat, corn, and soy. Since the mother was still nursing, in order to test the effects of a restricted diet on Emma's skin, both mother and daughter would need to completely avoid these foods for a few months.

I suggested that it might help to add some targeted nutritional support for Emma's skin. We used a liquid form of vitamin A in low doses, flaxseed oil, and some zinc. Her mother devised a way to dissolve these ingredients together and sneak them in with juice.

Thinking that Emma's gut might also benefit from support, we added liquid digestive enzymes with meals and snacks, to help her fully break down her food. She also took low daily doses of powdered probiotics and glutamine to help her gut cells cope with the stress they were presumably under.

Emma's mother worked hard to administer this regimen. One month went by without change, and then another. Both were growing more tired and crabby. It felt like failure.

But by the third month of her integrative care plan, Emma, now eighteen months old, toddled in with cheeks smooth and rosy for the first time in nine months. Mom's eyes were sparkling. The bags were gone. She was getting her life back, and it was on her terms, not the terms of the dermatologist or the steroid.

When I asked how she was doing, she flashed a wide smile. "Much better. Look—I have goose bumps," she said, showing me her arm.

"That makes two of us."

If you were there, you might have had goose bumps too.

A pastor friend once referred to emotional goose bumps as a form of "divine influx," a kind of mind-body phase transition that resonates throughout the system with a message akin to "This pleases God." A physician-acupuncturist friend referred to them as "healing moments," phase changes that reorient a body-mind toward wellness. All I know is that they were rare before I began using an integrative clinical mind-set, and now they're commonplace.

A case like this makes evidence-based sticklers bristle. There is no way to tease apart the relative contributions of food elimi-nation from dietary supplementation. Emma could have just grown out of it. Conventional colleagues would press the ques-tion, "Where's the data?" In response, I would quote Norman Cousins (1915-1990), "Never underestimate the value of a study whose number of subjects is one." This would hold them off while I got busy scrubbing the medical literature for studies supporting what I was doing.

I often found data where they weren't looking; it was in for-eign medical journals, the scientifically refereed naturopathic lit-erature, or buried deep in our own conventional journals. Yet few studies were of the kind that satisfies the modern judge of medical evidence. So why was I feeling pulled to a way of practice whose evidence base was weak by conventional standards? The answer was, and remains, that the clinical systems biology approach to chronic illness won my loyalty by the way it helped me produce desired results for my patients.

There was something wrong about being drilled by col-leagues to produce randomized controlled data when my practice data showed that two-thirds of my patients with persistent, unexplained symptoms of chronic illness were reporting moderate to major improvement within three to nine months of an integrative care plan based on a clinical systems biology approach.

The conventional approach to judging the quality of medical evidence discounts the use of inductive logic in sorting out the next right thing to do for a given patient. Using customary filters on medical evidence, the road stops where controlled studies are nowhere to be found. Because insurers are less like to reward doctors for inducing their way to solutions that work, patients with medically unexplained illnesses are left at the end of the road. The physician rushes back to the land where properly controlled studies dictate what should be done for the patient in the next room.

Inductive logic is a problem-solving tool; it reasons from historical and physical facts to larger patterns that hold power to explain the nature of a patient's health problems. When the patient's problems are chronic and complex, it takes longer to ride inductive logic to a conclusion because there is more territory to cover in terms of history, examination, and laboratory investigation. But to succeed in our health care sector these days, most medical practices cannot skimp on their need for speed. Insurers and their allies will keep seeing to that, using your money.

The integrative doctor is blessed with the opportunity to use inductive logic to craft a care plan uniquely fitted to a patient with persistent chronic problems—and free to make judgments without significant p-values to back them up. A p-value is the probability that a given study result occurred by chance. In medicine, most studies aren't taken seriously unless their p-values are less than 0.01, meaning that the result found would be caused by chance in less than one in one hundred cases. A dependence on p-values is what led to Emma's prescription for a more potent steroid. But as Dr. John Ioannidis has shown, most of the studies that post significant p-values cannot be replicated over time and turn out to be false and misleading.

Integrative care plans commonly ask both patient and physician to tolerate more than a fair share of ambiguity. But it is a tolerable price to pay for a care plan that addresses the multiple dimensions of *your* unique chronic illness experience. The trail of inductive logic should be retraceable in the integrative physician's medical record entries. Instead of basing judgment on the findings of an RCT, the functional medicine doctor may set up a trial and error study where you are the only subject of interest, and the methods used include systematic observation, reassessment, and adjustment as needed to move you closer to functional restoration. This is how the clinical systems biologist generates happy results for patients where usual and customary care has failed. Relying on randomized, controlled trials to decide how to approach your health problems may move you closer to treatment goals; the trouble is, the goals aren't always yours—they are often those of the health insurer, and of the providers that put the insurer's policies ahead of patient interests.

Shared problem solving aimed at root causes, emphasizing a broader understanding of how living systems work and what natural therapies can support them, just makes sense. Use an integrative clinical mind-set to find better answers and you may discover its surprising power to attain deeply hoped-for results despite challenges that seemed insurmountably complex.

A clinical systems biology approach creates the kind of medical care process and results that health consumers are looking for and that many doctors wish to provide. This radically empirical approach to medical knowledge management and translation into the language of whole person care deserves a seat at the table of medical education. It is part and parcel of the informational literacy that patients should expect from their doctors.

I took the goose bump exchange with Emma's mother as a sign that I was on the right path, one that promised to reveal a powerful approach to healing if I followed it with an open mind. I came to see that there is more going on in the human bodymind than the conventional mind-set allows, or has time for. I'm convinced to this day that the most insidious form of quackery is the closed professional mind.

With advances in systems biology research, it is becoming increasingly clear that the most powerful medicine in the world exists within you, in the form of healing systems based on a metabolic problem-solving wisdom that has evolved over millennia. An integrative clinical mind-set is ideally positioned to help you tap into the power of this healing wisdom.

With rare exceptions, being diagnosed with a disease does not mean that your system has lost its power to heal. But your ability to restore metabolic balance will almost always depend on what framework is being used to assess what's going on.

An integrative clinical mind-set seeks multiple ways to leverage a person's systems into metabolic balance. It emphasizes healthy lifestyle changes and natural therapies, self-care education, and cautious use of drugs and procedures when warranted. But there's more. An integrative clinical mind-set can also be used to support the health and wellness of living systems at other levels.

An integrative clinical mind-set is now being used to link disciplines in physics, biology, psychology, sociology, medicine, ecology, and economics, forming knowledge intersections that never before existed.

The integration of scientific disciplines is happening because it puts humanity in a better position to address signs of chronic illness within the Earth system. For example, the loss of biodiversity through climate change, wild habitat shrinkage, soil erosion, air and water contamination, and species over-harvesting are being studied as a set of problems whose solutions will require an integration of knowledge across many disciplines.

Retaining biodiversity means not losing genetic diversity, thereby preserving nature's degrees of freedom for maintaining balanced ecosystems. The mainstream medical profession may be slower to adopt an integrative mind-set than the rest of mainstream academia because its cash flow channels are ossified into place. But with the regulations of the Affordable Care Act well underway, the cracks in the health care sector's cash flow channels are starting to show. Crises in the health care sector are opportunities for integrative medicine.

Mayo, Harvard, Duke, UCSF, UCLA, Georgetown, Arizona, Illinois, Maryland, Wisconsin, MD Anderson, and dozens of other prestigious schools, medical centers, have established programs that expose medical students and residents to the principles and methods used by various practitioners with demonstrable skills in the realm of integrative medicine. Among the 160 American schools awarding MD or DO degrees, thirty percent, are members of the Consortium of Academic Health Centers for Integrative Medicine.

There are reasons why adoption is slow. Integrative medicine programs face two problems establishing themselves within academic medical center habitats: they don't generate as much revenue per square foot compared to plentiful alternatives, and they buck the system to varying degrees. Specialists may view an integrative medicine program as a threat. They've been known to show up at meetings to ask with furrowed brows, "You're going to treat what we treat doing what?"

To be fair, leading an academic medical center through turbulent times is not an easy job. Why take on the political risk and invite medical staff battles that, in an already difficult business and political climate, may be un-winnable? For medical staff who are used to being paid for the volume of services they provide, the change to being paid for the value produced by your services will be difficult to manage. For the integrative physician, getting paid on the value created by your results is a welcome change. Bring it on.

As an integrative approach to the life sciences develops a track record for demonstrating more problem-solving power, sophisticated health consumers will be hot on the trail of the health care implications of integrative problem solving. If their favorite academic medical center has yet to adopt a stance toward integrative medicine, it won't stop the sophisticated health consumer from looking elsewhere for expertise in this area.

What many consumers will have trouble discerning is how to choose whom to consult within the loosely organized realm of integrative medicine. Modalities such as acupuncture, homeopathy, herbal medicines, massage, subtle energy methods, and mind-body techniques all have their place, but what knowledge base can organize such skills and traditions into a coherent, value-creating whole?

Based on my experience, the answer to this question is functional medicine—an in-depth, personalized, results-driven

approach to medical care that gives integrative medicine a science-based core. Functional medicine runs on a clinical systems
biology engine whose fuel is research from the life sciences.

Chronic illness research has reached the point where we can
finally say that systems biology evidence doesn't merely inform
an integrative clinical mind-set—it *requires* it. Conventional and
alternative clinical mind-sets are too one dimensional in their
approaches to what counts as knowledge to fully translate systems
biology evidence into health wisdom and wellness results

Because of the way PubMed, PLoS, Google, Wikipedia, and
other Web-based tools have helped democratize access to scientific research findings, the days of special interest spin are drawing
to a close. Science is one of several tools needed in our search for
wisdom about health and healing—not the only tool. Consumers
know this. They will not be satisfied with spin, subterfuge or patent oversimplification of the physician's task.

The good news is that a future worth wanting and creating—
a future of health, wellness, and sustainability—is visible on the
horizon. It is a future that will turn seemingly insurmountable
challenges into decipherable problems whose solutions can lead
us to deeply hoped-for results.

To get there, all we have to do is value the health and functional integrity of greater wholes as if our future depends on it.

Tending to the Integrity
of Greater Wholes

◇◇◇◇◇◇◇◇◇◇◇◇◇◇◇◇◇◇◇◇◇◇◇◇◇◇◇◇◇◇◇◇◇

Part of the genius of Cervantes' *Don Quixote* was that he made inscrutable the dividing line between reality-based thinking and madness. Quixote had crazy ideas, yet we suspected he wasn't thoroughly mad. Moments of clarity would break through, as when he protested, "Too much sanity may be madness, and maddest of all, to see life as it is and not as it should be!"

In thinking how to go about organizing a grass roots quest for health and sustainability, we should explore what kind of philosophy should guide us, expecting that time and again on such a quest will we be asked to choose life as it is, or life as it ought to be.

Quixote had the good fortune of having a rational and faithful companion at his side. Sancho Panza was his foil, his prod, and his open-minded interpreter—in a way, his integrative clinical mind-set. Humanity needs an open-minded interpreter—a rational and faithful companion able to wield an integrative clinical mind-set.

As we strive for the clearest possible understanding of how nature works, we must also be humble with regard to the limits of what we can know about our ultimate origins and purpose. The issue that most frustrates our contemplations of where we come from and where we should be going is the problem of evil. We can't ignore the stench of it.

Sir Edmund Burke (1729–1797) once said, "All that is needed for the triumph of evil is that good men do nothing." In the *Tao Te Ching*, Lao Tzu wrote, "Give evil nothing to oppose and it will disappear by itself." So which is it? Are we to oppose evil or ignore it?

Google's mission statement—"Don't be evil"— asks those who would lead to resist embodying evil. It may not be the best we can do, but active self-restraint would close some of the portals through which evil snakes into the world and into our lives. There would be less evil to oppose or ignore if we took our personal and corporate responsibilities more seriously.

If evil is like a virus that won't go away, we might at least work on chasing it into a dormant state. The problem of evil can thus be viewed as a clinical problem: How can we hound evil into dormancy, and how should we metabolize the suffering caused by evil when it activates?

The challenge is steep because, as our species evolved, our ancestors developed instincts to lie, cheat, steal, hate, abuse, injure, and kill as a way to survive—instincts that stir in us still. Survival instinct cannot simply be erased, but education and leadership by example can help us gain better control over biological drives that might otherwise foster evildoing. It would also help if most people could feel they have an equal opportunity to survive and live a secure and dignified life. That would require more than education and leadership by example—it would require cultural change.

Our challenge is to find personal and communal goals that freely align from one culture to another. A goal that might pull cultures toward alignment is our shared need to promote the functional integrity of greater wholes—starting with the greater whole that is you, and moving on to include the greater wholes that are your family, your community, your society, and the entire world of living systems. Success in a cross-cultural quest for health and sustainability will fortify our efforts to fully make life what it ought to be.

How do we know that human nature and its genetically driven biological urges can be reshaped? We know this because adapting our drives to fit changing environmental circumstances is what has gotten us this far in the evolutionary process. The issue boils down to how fast we can adapt in an age where we depend less on our genes and more on our ideas and our ability to change our cultures and social institutions.

Inspiration has a long track record of motivating positive changes in behavior without the help of financial or material incentives or threats of violence. As major sources of inspiration, spiritual and artistic works are great allies in our quest for a developing a positive human relationship to the world.

When Stevie Wonder questions evil in his song of the same name, his laments go unanswered, but the way they're sung is enough to make listeners care about loosening evil's grip on our lives. Artistic brilliance inspires the will to change by a more congenial route than political ideology. Virtuoso artistic performances reach across the aisle—they can shrink political divides, albeit briefly. Virtuoso skills will be needed on the path to health and sustainability. Survival summons endless variations on virtuosity.

Spiritual and artistic traditions are allies in the human quest for health and wellness because they spread joy and inspiration across cultural boundaries, reminding us that we're not so different. Democrats and Republicans are equally moved by a beautifully arranged, well-sung national anthem, but as soon as it is over they resume their hostilities. This gives us the impression that the quest for power defies all else, including beauty, awe, health, and sustainability. This may be more a statement about the corrupting lure of political power than a statement about a permanent flaw in human nature.

With inspiration comes a desire for ethically responsible action within one's sphere of influence. Serving the integrity of the greater whole through ethically responsible action emerges not just as a fitting project for each human being, but as a fitting way to serve the interests of the greater whole. Without knowing quite why, we are called to build a dignified response to the creative force that acted first and allowed us to enter the picture.

We are thrust into the role of pathfinders for life. The Earth system is the sphere of influence for our species. We're not yet sure what kind of influence it will take to move our cultures toward health and sustainability. We suspect that winning hearts and minds is a necessary but insufficient way of changing the world. Deeper, higher forms of organization and integration will be required.

We're beginning to sense that somewhere in our future is a shared path to our most sacred ideals, a path that will lead us toward wiser care of our own bodyminds and wiser care of the developing bodymind of humanity. We are now the dominant presence whose impact is both fair and foul, tinged with a drive for excellence and a capacity for evil. The recurrence of evildoing is like a persistent, medically unexplained symptom. When usual and customary care fails to solve the problem, we turn to a clinical systems biology approach managed by an integrative clinical mindset, and we learn that some of our beliefs and lifestyles will need to change.

The meanings you draw from the pages to come will reflect your own patterns of belief and interpretation, shaped by what history has revealed to you. The meaning that you take away will bear the stamp of your own faith and political traditions, your own systems for making sense of information, and your own ideologies for what counts as wisdom and as reason for action.

The universe keeps unfolding. New data keep streaming into our ways of viewing the world. These data include findings from science, interpretations from theology and religion, creative expressions from the realms of artistic imagination, the networking capabilities of social media, and much more. In this integrated stream of information, meaning seems to have no top or bottom, no inside or out—yet as globalization proceeds on its precarious path, we can feel it pointing us in a particular direction: the way of health and sustainability.

It's as if the evolving bodymind of humanity wants to organize itself around principles of health and wellness, and this growing, collective desire among the world's people is what will finally place an ethical imperative at the front and center of our personal and institutional lives. We can see how true it is that we're all in this together, yet our thoughts easily stray to the politics of fear, where sustainability is a function of security, defense, and a survival instinct that makes us ready to kill or be killed. The politics of fear can exploit our insecurities and draw our attention away from finding sustainable solutions to our social, economic, and environmental problems.

The Internet has emerged as a tool that can shed light on almost anything. But on the Web, brilliance, laughter, and inspiration compete for our attention against evil, vice, and utter nonsense. The most precious resource you can share within your sphere of influence is your attention.

There is growing potential for an influential coalition of wise consumers whose motto is, "Aim high before you buy"—that is, a desire to reward those companies, markets, and elected representatives that take the long view, going the extra mile to make the world a healthier, safer, more dignified home for our children's children. Because money talks, allied consumers might help us find what entrenched ideologues cannot: real solutions to complex problems.

Slowly but surely we feel the collective wish to end the kind of thinking that divides the world into "us vs. them." The politics of fear works if your goal is to get elected. If the goal is to get selected—by nature and perhaps by God—the politics of fear must be transformed into a politics of health and sustainability.

Despite the diversity and conflict that appear on the human surface, deep down we are the same: we all know pain, we all want to live dignified lives, and, if we take the time to think it through, we want to do what's within our means to secure a healthier, more stable Earth system.

We are not complete novices on the subject of environmental conservation. We're accumulating scientific knowledge on the subject at a brisk clip, and there are clear signs of the interdisciplinary integration needed to translate what we're learning into effective conservation plans. Most important, there are signs of passionate commitment to the cause.

Eric Chivian is the founder of the Center for Health and the Global Environment, and an assistant professor of psychiatry at Harvard Medical School. In 1980 he co-founded International Physicians for the Prevention of Nuclear War, an organization that won the Nobel Peace Prize in 1985. He educates physicians and the public on the health value of environmental conservation. He is a leading example of what it is like to be a passionate steward of the Earth system.

The same can be said of Aaron Bernstein, a pediatric hospitalist on the faculty of Harvard Medical School, and a research associate at the Center for Heath and the Global Environment. Chivian and Bernstein co-edited the 2008 scientific compilation *Sustaining Life: How Human Health Depends on Biodiversity*. Bernstein was the lead author of this work, which, all told, involved the efforts of almost three hundred people.

One of the many notable things about this effort is how much it both illuminates and inspires its readers. An excerpt from the book's preface speaks to why they sought so many helping hands in completing this project:

> Scientists with expertise in a wide range of disciplines, from industrialized and developing countries alike, have been involved in putting this book together. We have done so because we are convinced that it can help people understand that human beings are an integral part of Nature, and that our health depends ultimately on the health of its species and on the natural functioning of its ecosystems. We have done so because all of us hope that our efforts will help guide policy

makers in developing innovative and equitable policies based on sound science that will effectively preserve biodiversity and promote human health for generations to come. And we have done so, finally, because we all believe that life on Earth is sacred and that we must never give up on trying to preserve it, and because we all share the conviction that once people recognize how much is at stake with their health and lives, and with the health and lives of their children, they will do everything in their power to protect the global environment.

The following is an excerpt from the book's dedication:

We dedicate this book to the millions of plant, animal, and microbial species we share this small planet with, and to our own species, *Homo sapiens*, who first walked on Earth some 195,000 years ago and struggled to survive over the millennia to become the magnificent and extraordinarily powerful beings we are today. May we have the wisdom, and the love for our children and all children to come, to use that power to save the indescribably beautiful and precious gift we have been given.

Edward O. Wilson, the father of modern sociobiology and a leading voice for would-be stewards of living systems, has this to say in the book's foreword:

Ecologists have long used the metaphor of the canary in the mine to caution humanity. Like the delicate little birds once carried into coal mines following explosions or fires in order to detect poisonous gases, some sensitive plants and animals around us, by virtue of their sickness and dying, give early warning of dangerous changes in our common environment. The masterful presentations in *Sustaining Life* document beyond reasonable doubt that we are at risk of becoming a canary in today's world. In myriad ways humanity is linked to the millions of other species on this planet. What concerns them equally concerns us. The more we ignore our common health and welfare, the greater are the many threats to our own species. The better we understand and the more we rationally manage our relationship with the rest of life, the greater the guarantee of our own safety and quality of life.

As a young boy, Wilson was blinded in his right eye when the dorsal fin spine of a fish he had caught punctured his eye. Despite this rude introduction to nature, Wilson, now in his mid-eighties, has received over one hundred awards for his research, writing, and project development efforts in the areas of social evolution, biodiversity, and environmental conservation.

In his foreword to *Sustaining Life*, he acknowledges that most people are aware of the threats posed by pollution, ozone depletion, and habitat destruction—but they are not as aware of how this already affects human well-being:

> The reason is the prevailing worldview that health is largely an internal matter for our species, and, with the exception of domesticated species and pathogenic microorganisms, the rest of life is something else...The mismanagement and destruction of species and ecosystems ongoing around the world mindlessly, and needlessly, lower the quality of the planet's natural resources, destabilize the physical environment, and can hasten the spread of human infectious diseases and the invasive enemies of the crops and forests on which our lives depend.

Wilson also comments on the subject of mining the bodymind wisdom of other species:

Bioprospecting, the exploration of diversity in order to open its mother lode of new pharmaceuticals, is still largely neglected and rudimentary. Little attempt has been made to utilize natural biodiversity to enhance public health.

Chivian and Bernstein offer plenty of examples that illustrate what biodiversity loss could mean to human health. One in particular stands out: the story of the gastric brooding frogs, *Rheobatrachus silus* and *Rheobatrachus vitellinus*.

Discovered in pristine sections of the Australian rainforest in the 1980s, gastric brooders are the only frogs to raise their young in their stomachs. The female swallows fertilized eggs, and only when the hatchlings reach the tadpole stage does she regurgitate them into the water.

Research teams took a serious interest in how the eggs become young tadpoles without being harmed by the mother's stomach acid or being propelled into her small intestine along with the bugs she's eaten. Analysis suggested that stomach chemicals secreted by the mother or by the young gave hope for a novel treatment for people with peptic ulcer disease and gastroesophageal reflux disorder.

Doctors and patients would welcome a treatment that avoided the trade-offs involved in the chronic use of potent antacids, whose adverse effects include irritable bowel symptoms, low magnesium levels, and bone density loss, with an increased rate of hip fracture in older patients.

We'll never know what chemicals allow gastric brooding frogs to pull off their one-of-a-kind amphibian gestation method, because they're now extinct—gone, along with their genome that went back some 350 million years.

One third of the world's 6,155 amphibian species are endangered, and roughly two percent are on the verge of extinction. Their genomes hold the secrets of how to survive their early months underwater and their adult lives on land. Chemicals isolated from frogs serve an unusually wide range of functions and show great medical potential, ranging from pain and blood pressure control to cartilage repair and tumor suppression.

Frogs, salamanders, and caecilians are especially sensitive to habitat loss or habitat alteration by invasive species, global warming and increased ultraviolet B radiation exposure, and perhaps also to parasites associated with poor water quality. Their increased exposure to pollution is of escalating concern.

Atrazine, an herbicide commonly used to control weeds that would otherwise steal nutrients from corn, soy, and other crops, is in the lineup of perpetrators suspected of increasing amphibian extinction threats to levels higher than anything seen in the prior fossil record. Atrazine is but one of many thousands of industrial chemicals suspected of causing adverse biological effects within living systems.

The question under dispute is whether or not atrazine causes reproductive abnormalities in various frog species. Environmental scientists and industry-sponsored experts have been trying to settle this dispute for decades. The result is a classic fight over a key principle in systems biology and environmental conservation: *absence of proof is not proof of absence.*

Recent research now indicates with a high degree of confidence that atrazine demasculinizes male gonads, not just in frogs, but also in male vertebrates of all kinds—fish, frogs, reptiles, and mammals like us.

A leader in this area of environmental health research is Tyrone B. Hayes, a professor of biology at the University of California at Berkeley and a member of their Department of Integrative Biology. In a study released by the *Journal of Steroid Biochemistry and Molecular Biology*, Hayes and nineteen other colleagues have shown that atrazine not only has these feminizing effects on male vertebrates, but that the evidence claiming to prove it meets the stringent Hill criteria for establishing cause-effect relationships between variables in complex biological systems.

To establish a cause and effect relationship between, say, a potentially hazardous chemical and a particular adverse health effect in certain types of organisms or species within a given eco-system, the following nine Hill criteria must be met:

1. Strength (the probability of being wrong is low).

2. Consistency (when the cause is present, the effect reliably occurs).

3. Specificity (a particular cause produces a particular effect).

4. Temporality (the cause reliably precedes the effect).

5. Biological gradient (if the cause is amplified, so is the effect).

6. Plausibility (the cause-effect relationship makes sense).

7. Coherence (there are no obvious flaws in the logic used to support the claim).

8. Experiment (the relationship holds up under experimental conditions).

9. Analogy (there are instances of such relationships elsewhere in biology).

The British medical statistician Austin Bradford Hill (1897–1991) proposed these criteria, which formed the basis of modern epidemiological research and went on to form the standard for medical research in general.

An atrazine debate sideshow involves a character assassination contest between professor Hayes and Syngenta, the company that manufactures most of the world's atrazine. In this ongoing feud, Hayes has at times donned the persona of an e-mail rapper, quoting lyrics from hip-hop songs in exchanges with representatives of Syngenta.

The trash-talking e-mails may have been unprofessional, but they added spice and attracted journalistic interest that rarely covers such disputes. Most discussions involving environmental controversies lack the zip needed to catch public attention. In this case, Syngenta's strategy of shooting arrows while playing the victim may backfire, as it only drew more media and legal attention to the issue. Lawsuits against Syngenta include fifteen by water providers in Illinois seeking $350 million to help remove atrazine from drinking water.

Since the 1970s Illinois has also seen a steep decline in the population of its cricket frogs (*Acris crepitans*), once the most common amphibians in the state. As Bernstein notes in *Sustaining Life*, pollution is the leading reason for this decline.

A team of researchers compared the gonads of over eight hundred museum specimens of cricket frogs collected from specific Illinois locations between 1852 and 2001 and stored in sixteen museums statewide. Researchers discovered that signs of hermaphrodism (frog gonads showing features of testicular and ovarian anatomy at the same time) were found more often in a certain group of frogs. The results showed that the highest risk of intersex changes was found in frogs collected between 1946 and 1959, a period of major industrial growth when multipurpose polychlorinated biphenyls (PCBs) and the pesticide DDT were in peak production.

Researchers also found that the highest hermaphrodism risk occurred in frogs collected from the urbanized and heavily industrialized corridors in the northeastern portion of the state. This study offered clear evidence that hormonal disruption of reproductive function caused by exposure to persistent organic pollutants (POPs) likely accounted for the Illinois cricket frog's vanishing act.

The banning of DDT in 1972 and PCBs in 1979 resulted in decreased exposures to wildlife and correlates with rebounding population counts, including the steady recovery of the country's bald eagle population from its low point of only four hundred nesting pairs in the early 1970s.

Yet dozens of other POPs continue to find their way into our air, water, soils, and vegetation. In 2001, when Hayes reported atrazine-induced hermaphrodism in leopard frogs exposed to only 0.1 parts per billion, he ignited the controversy with Syngenta, a company whose spokespeople keep insisting that atrazine is not a proven hormone disrupter despite solid evidence to the contrary.

Some question Hayes' decision to inject hip-hop styling into his ongoing debate with Syngenta concerning the health hazards of atrazine. Whatever the public relations and court battles decide, the evidence is in, and as far as that goes, Hayes' scientific integrity is not in question. There's more than money at stake as this drama unfolds. What's really at stake is the integrity of our species.

Back to the elder statesman of biodiversity, Professor Wilson, closing his foreword to *Sustaining Life*:

> The shift in worldview recommended by the authors of *Sustaining Life* is predicated on the increasingly obvious principle that humanity, having evolved as part of the web of life, remains enmeshed within it. We do not float above the biosphere in some higher spiritual or techno-scientific plane. For many reasons, not least our own wellbeing, we need to take better care of the rest of life. Biodiversity will pay off in every sphere of human life, from medical to economic, from our collective security to our spiritual fulfillment.

We are only beginning to accept that we are pathfinders seeking relief from our own misadventures. Our minds are opening. We are growing up and finding ourselves. We are seeking a more fitting way to respond to our shared cosmic circumstance, uncertain about the source of our being, frustrated by the problem of evil, and not sure about how much we want to cooperate with each other and with the living systems that have sponsored us this far.

In the ceaseless jockeying for position among the species on Earth, we find ourselves ahead of the pack, *de facto* pathfinders, stewards in the making, lacking the necessary skills but showing signs of an angry eagerness to learn how to tend to the integrity of the greater whole. This eagerness subsides when we learn that our path to health and sustainability will require some self-imposed rethinking of our worldviews.

From Genesis to Responsibility

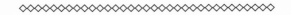

You possess one of the most impressive gene regulation systems the universe has ever produced—as far as we can tell. There may be other twisted spirals of genes elsewhere in the cosmos, busy reproducing themselves, evolving into organisms, developing consciousness and intelligence, and doing their best to figure out what life is about, and what it is they are meant to be and to do. For all we know, there are living systems elsewhere in the cosmos that have evolved to aspire to higher purposes, only to falter and fade out.

A full copy of your gene regulation system can be found inside your nucleated cells. This system manages a micro-universe of biochemical operations every second and can do so for decades before succumbing to the natural forces of disease or age-related disintegration.

Our species is equipped with a reproduction system so efficient that by the end of this century some ten billion of us could inhabit a planet whose terrestrial landscape is increasingly less wild and more "developed" by the geniuses now governing the business of the planet.

A patch of wild land is formally defined as ten thousand square kilometers populated by few people and with habitat comprising ninety percent or more native species of plants and animals. Only forty-three percent of the world's landmass currently meets this definition of "wild." Much of this land is considered too harsh for human habitation and would require substantial infrastructure development to support a decent standard of living. When there are ten billion of us, we'll see what we can do about that.

When it comes to gene regulation prowess, we humans have no rival. When it comes to adverse impact on the Earth's eco-systems, again we have no rival. Are we incapable of preventing nature's best genetic program from becoming nature's worst social program?

Every organism and social system on Earth represents a set of patterns and processes whose interdependent parts take on a uniquely complex identity as a whole. These complex patterns and processes of interdependence seem to develop new computational rule sets on the fly, without gaining permission from the slow-moving natural selection process. Evolution, as it turns out, includes the sudden and unpredictable emergence of new patterns and processes of interdependence.

This ability of complex systems to suddenly emerge into states that contain new laws and properties is challenging the orthodox theory that biodiversity is purely a product of chance, natural selection, and deep stretches of time. Living systems on Earth have been transforming information into physical complexity at an accelerating pace going on four billion years now. We should never be surprised to learn that reality turns out to be more complex than we thought.

In *Programming the Universe,* Seth Lloyd explains how he and his colleague, the late Heinz Pagels (1939–1988), came to think about complexity. They began with a simple definition first proposed by mathematician Charles Bennett, which related complexity to a trade-off between the information a system had gathered and the effort it took to gather it.

According to Bennett's scheme, complex systems that gathered the most information with the least effort had the most *logical depth.* Pagels felt that this definition was mathematically sound but not physical enough, so he and Lloyd jointly devised the concept of *thermodynamic depth.*

Logical depth means information processing power and efficiency; thermodynamic depth means physical organization, power, and efficiency. The greater the logical and thermodynamic depth within a complex system, the more that system can oppose and stall the disintegrating forces of nature.

Simple systems, such as a rock or a desk, are thermodynamically shallow. "But," writes Lloyd, "intricate, structured systems such as living systems, required a huge investment of useful bits [of information] over billions of years to assemble and are thermodynamically deep."

Among all the organisms ever found in the Earth system, none surpasses the logical and thermodynamic depth of the human bodymind.

From the standpoint of an integrative clinical mind-set, the logical and thermodynamic depth of the Earth's living systems as a whole represents a vast storage network for bodymind wisdom. Within this network, biodiversity loss involves species extinction.

Think of extinction as being like permanently deleting a priceless work from the hard disk of life. You never know what cures or solutions are lost in the process.

The functional integrity of your bodymind depends on your capacity to manage information, energy, and substance. In this reservoir of bodymind functionality you will find the most powerful medicine in the world.

In *Complexity: A Guided Tour*, Melanie Mitchell observes that all complex systems hold these intriguing properties in common:

1. They consist of networked components capable of self-organizing behaviors.

2. They generate and make use of information and signaling systems from both internal and external environments.

3. They adapt by changing their behavior in ways that improve their chances of survival or success.

Self-organization, self-regulation, and adaptation are important properties because they're needed for living systems to defy the second law of thermodynamics, which states that the ability of energy to accomplish work always decays toward zero, to a state of maximum entropy, or disorganization. This means that the only thing standing in the way of a total collapse of living systems—including the living system that is you—is logical and thermodynamic depth. To put it more simply, nature builds things that successfully resist nature's own tendency to disintegrate them. How did this happen?

The answer is found in what a group of university-based teachers call *big history*—a science-based multidisciplinary history of the universe from the Big Bang to now. David Christian is perhaps the most notable contributor to the telling of this history, as recounted in his book *Maps of Time: An Introduction to Big History.*

In this book, Christian presents a "single, grand, intelligible narrative" of the cosmos, beginning with the Big Bang some 13.7 billion years ago. A ten-million-degree furnace eventually gave rise to subatomic particles, and then to the atoms hydrogen and helium. As these atoms coalesced into stars, supernovas kicked out a variety of additional, more complex atomic structures: carbon, nitrogen, oxygen, and so on.

Rocky planets formed, rich in the elements that we list on the periodic table. Planets with reservoirs of water or other liquids sponsored the random mixing of these elements. On Earth, "Goldilocks" conditions (environmental states that were "just right") gave rise to amino acids, sugars, fats, and nucleic acids. Goldilocks conditions then led to single-celled protobacterial forms, and then to more complex single-celled creatures, the eukaryotes. These more complex cells contained specialized subunits called organelles, including energy-producing mitochondria. Eukaryotes enclosed their genes within a nucleus. These genes provided a template for reproducing the proteins and biochemical interactions needed to sustain their cell types over multiple generations.

Eukaryotic gene mixing began the long process of the natural selection of genes that conferred survival advantages to their host creatures, which led to the first multi-celled organisms. By 195,000 years ago, our lineage, the great and wonderful *Homo sapiens*, appeared. This smartest of monkeys developed language and gave rise to increasingly elaborate cultures, warehouses of learning and ways of managing knowledge, values, beliefs, and traditions. Cultures became ideal incubators for new technologies.

The host of complex living systems on Earth organized them-selves into ecosystems that have thus far avoided reaching a Mars-like state of entropy. But in the very short span of three hun-dred years, human technology has become the major threat to the health and sustainability of a growing number of the Earth's ecosystems. Thus, big history appears to be on a long stroll from genesis to responsibility. Without a sense of responsibility for the health of living systems, the rulers of Earthville may find them-selves on a mad dash to survive their own ignorance.

Ecosystems are commonly pictured as landscapes—prairies, highlands, wetlands, islands, and so on. The truth is, ecosystems exist at every level in the hierarchy of natural systems, from the microbial ecosystems of the mammalian bowel to the more tra-ditional large-scale networks of wild habitats teeming with life.

When these interdependent living systems lose integrative strength, their logical and thermodynamic depth recedes to shal-lower levels, enabling chronic illness to take hold because the sys-tem as a whole is losing degrees of freedom for self-regulating its way out of trouble. Just as your bodymind can lose degrees of freedom for figuring things out on its own, so can an ecosystem lose degrees of freedom for sustaining itself as a balanced whole.

Instead of working on ways to help your systems reintegrate their ability to generate self-healing solutions to complex prob-lems, the busy doctor prescribes a drug, hoping that blocking a receptor or inhibiting an enzyme in this pathway or that will solve enough of the problem to slow the pace at which your health is getting worse. In the case of a simple bladder infection the right drug can help your body catch up and heal. In the case of chronic multidimensional health problems, drugs alone may help keep you out of the hospital, but they will not lead you to the promised land of health and wellness.

Complex chronic health problems call for root-level solutions—care plans that carry more logical and thermodynamic depth than a list of drugs. They require plans that permeate more deeply and widely into your bodily systems; plans that start with lifestyle medicine and natural therapies and turn to medications only when justified; plans aimed at helping you repair the onboard systems responsible for restoring the functions you have lost.

Whether the interdependent parts are the metabolic systems of your body or the cultural systems of our clashing civilizations, degrees of freedom for maintaining health and sustainability will likely keep slipping the longer we rely on simple solutions to complex problems.

We invest billions in drug development with the idea that our creations can outsmart nature or do it one better. At times this conceit works amazingly well, but not often enough to warrant the huge investments. Drug companies are pulling out of formerly attractive chronic disease markets because they recognize that chronic disease equations are too complex to submit to simple drug solutions. This creates an opening for a clinical systems biology approach.

Of course we can't prevent all diseases and no one makes it out alive. This fact feeds our existential anxiety about the inevitability of suffering, death, and the evil that lurks around the bend. Reality is a harsh stage for life and the wonderment of being. Cold reality makes us feel guilty and condemned for even being alive. What positive meaning can we draw from the flow of our existence, and what power does positive meaning have to help us conquer our anxieties about fate, death, guilt, meaninglessness, and doubt?

We turn to science, mysticism, philosophy, and religion in search of answers and succor. Our deepest existential anxieties stem from having no recourse but to accept that our own being must cross-fade into non-being. This fact gives rise to the fear that from non-being there is no exit.

We have heard from science about the big history of the cosmos, which offers answers but only to a degree. The net result is little balm for existential suffering.

The mystic wisdom of the Buddhist tradition offers practical help when it comes to coping with our discontents. As Buddhist teacher Ajahn Amaro writes in the compendium, *The Mind's Own Physician,* "One of the epithets Guatama Buddha (563 BC-483 BC) acquired over the years was "doctor of the world." A reason for this is that "the central insight and framework that he taught, known as the Four Noble Truths," can be "cast in the formulation of classical Indian medical diagnosis."

From this perspective, Buddhism becomes a clinical wisdom tradition in that it concerns itself with personal evaluation and care planning. The First Noble truth is to elicit a clear description of the symptom—the suffering or state of dissatisfaction that is being experienced by the individual. The Second Noble Truth is to understand the inner causes of the symptom. The Third Noble Truth is to establish a prognosis for healing the inner causes of the symptom. The Fourth Noble Truth is to determine the best method by which to heal the inner wounds that are causing the symptom.

Buddhist methods focus on self-understanding, mindfulness, meditation, and detaching from the fears and desires that cause us to suffer. They offer ways to deflect negative meaning using the courage of self-regulation. Buddhism stops short of guiding us on how to cope with the dark reality of the eternal contest between meaning and meaninglessness.

Philosophical existentialism addresses these deeper issues, most notably through the Stoics, from Socrates (469-399 BC), Seneca (4 BC-65 AD), and Epictetus (55-135 AD) in classical antiquity to Spinoza (1632-1677), Nietzsche (1844-1900), and Sartre (1905-1980) in the modern age. Stoicism takes the position that happiness follows those who can use their faculty of reason to tame their negative emotional responses to things.

Stoicism and Buddhism both summon self-regulation skills as a way to happiness. The Buddhist stops the reasoning mind in order to be fully present in the moment. By allowing negativity to go unprocessed by reason or the emotions, the Buddhist can achieve states of bliss simply by becoming one with being as it is, without judgment. By relying on rationality to talk down negative emotional responses to thoughts and perceptions, the Stoic contrives a path along which reason must pluck the weeds of emotional negativity, leaving only contentment.

Epictetus summarized the Stoic cure for anxiety when he said, "Come to believe that everything should unfold exactly as it does." Succeed at this, and you surely will find little to be unhappy about. Yet the Stoics did put reason to a higher purpose. The rational mind was given the task of finding the courage to be virtuous and wise in spite of the presence of evil, death, and suffering. And it takes reason and courage to metabolize your anxieties into wisdom and virtue. Socrates and Seneca each put this courage to its highest test when ordered by authorities to commit suicide for their impieties.

To Spinoza, courage powered the will to live. More precisely, courage powered the will to affirm and fulfill the purpose of one's being. To Nietzsche, life itself revealed the will to power, or, more precisely, the will to keep gaining strength. To a rational mind it is this will to power that yields the courage to affirm and fulfill the purpose of one's being. What's more, such power is able to let go of itself when the capacity to keep striving grows weak. When death comes calling, one can calmly make way for new life. Life will march on, seeking ways to gain strength. Death is a necessary step in life's ongoing battle with entropy, chaos, and non-being. The weak must give way to the strong.

All courage is born of confidence—of holding something within your self that possesses value worth affirming not only to yourself, but also to the culture in which you participate, and to the world in which you live, move, and have your being.

Sartre's nausea about our being condemned to be free was a contagion he caught from Nietzsche, who ran with the idea that meaning had run its course, a victim of modernity. Sartre took it a step farther in asserting that we have no Creator. In a world with no meaning, Sartre wrote, "Hell is other people." In a philosophical landscape this bleak, existential anxiety becomes nihilism, the smothering blanket that makes it harder than ever for us to summon the courage of confidence.

Nihilism is the product of the disproportionate tension between reality and the realization of our communal ideals; the difference between being as it is and being as it ought to be. It would take a will to power to throw off the weight of such despair and doubt. So where does that leave us?

The mystic teachings of Buddhism lead us to relief from suffering; they are content to let the universe ask the questions and supply its own the answers. The existentialists ask and answer their own philosophical questions and the answers grow drearier over time. As with scientific answers, philosophical answers are not all that therapeutic for the existential anxiety of the suffering soul. You are free to hire reason to tame your emotions, and science to reduce the value of your subjective experience, but see how happy and well it makes you feel.

We are not satisfied because the answers we are looking for as a species are clinical in nature—not the product of pure reason. We must accommodate meaning, and meaning is a product of both the objective and subjective dimensions of being human. Science and philosophical existentialism provide answers without comfort. Buddhism offers comfort without answers. Then comes religion offering comforting answers.

Paul Tillich (1886-1965) was a Christian theologian and existentialist. In his last major work, *The Courage to Be*, he comes to the conclusion that the anxiety created by the certainty of evil, death, and suffering, and by our resulting feelings of guilt, meaninglessness, and doubt, is most effectively treated when we accept that our being is redeemed by the grace of God. That is to say, when you accept that you are accepted in the grand scheme of things, anxiety subsides and you are free to be who you are meant to be. No more being shackled by your existential worries, fears, and desires. Through belief—accepting that you are accepted in spite of your flaws and weaknesses—you become best enabled to summon the existential courage it takes to move being from what it is toward what it ought to be.

The God idea is not so much asserted by Tillich as it is presented as a choice we are invited to make. In a worldview in which you are accepted, in which grace triumphs over death and the threatened total collapse of being into non-being, with your acceptance of the grace of God you have more courage to value and stand up for your self. With this courage you are called in response to such grace to help your culture radiate wisdom and virtue into its sphere of influence. The courage to be thereby moves beyond the will to power to shoulder responsibility for cultivating the flowering of all being within your sphere of influence. Courage is an act of taking ethical responsibility for how strength and power should be put to use.

Tillich finds the cure for existential anxiety in the idea of a loving God—the personal encounter between human being and divine being. The inspiration derived from such a personal encounter can carry courage beyond attempts to explain, deflect, or tame anxiety into a realm where the acceptance of divine love trumps fear and trust in divine providence removes doubt—even at times when hell is other people.

This contrasting of scientific, mystical, philosophical, and religious perspectives on how to deal with the genuinely nauseating reality of evil, death, and suffering will not settle our arguments about what to believe and how to live. Deciding what you should believe and how you should live is a personal decision. Deciding what our cultures should believe and how we should live together in a world with increasingly little space inhabitable by our species has become a fundamentally clinical decision. We need to summon the courage to adapt our cultures to support health and sustainability because it is the only responsible thing to do.

On the matter of death, we can say with confidence that when your thermodynamic depth decays to zero, you're dead—but you are not necessarily gone. That is because the logical depth that your presence brought into the world survives to some degree, not just in the memories of you kept by others, or the reminders of what you meant to them, but in the works you left behind and the ideas that they speak to. On the matter of evil, we should accept any route to the courage to do something about it. Ignoring evil is not part of a clinically sound care plan. On the matter of suffering, we can turn to the mystical or religious guides on the subject.

Once you die your genome is lost and gone forever, but your ideas can live on. Ideas worth keeping find their way into the wisdom traditions of humanity. Ideas not worth keeping have the potential to poison or sap the courage of our cultures to become better stewards of living systems.

Our cultures define our collective ways of being. They come in all different strengths and sizes, each one a coalescing around a set of shared values, beliefs, skills, and traditions. Great human civilizations have come and gone as the result of guns, germs, steel, corruption, incompetence, and evil. Our collective, cross-cultural ideas have yet to self-organize their way onto a path toward health and sustainability. We are responsible for the health and sustainability of living systems.

From an integrative clinical standpoint, health and sustainability seem to be calling upon all cultures to infuse their institutions and their individual adherents with an ethic of responsibility. The long arc of humanity reaches from the genesis of single-celled organisms to the dawning of ethical responsibility as a social organizing principle. Wisdom bearers over the generations could see this all along. Where are today's wisdom bearers?

To protect the depth of human genetic and cultural wisdom, the depth of our cultural and biodiversity, the human collective presence in the world must figure out how to institutionalize a sense of ethical responsibility. Our genetic code must be joined by a social code that promotes a more widespread commitment to a global ethic of responsibility.

Cultures don't take marching orders. They can't be told what to do. They appear highly resistant to change, even when the hearts and minds of the people are aligned and a few political and institutional leaders are on board with what needs to change. It takes more than that to change a culture.

To understand the mechanics of cultural change is to understand what it takes to change not just how power and influence flow through the system, but how courage and responsibility guide how power and influence ought to flow through the system.

Can we afford to wait for evidence-based cultural change research to point out the way to health and sustainability? Get real. The standard of care is letting us down not just in the health care sector, but virtually everywhere. We need to bring an integrative clinical mind-set to the task, in no small part because it requires us to tend to the integrity of greater wholes.

Our quest will force us to come to terms with the idea that the functional integrity of our species as a whole will depend on our willingness to limit some of our personal and corporate freedoms.

Freedom and
Functional Integration

◇◇◇◇◇◇◇◇◇◇◇◇◇◇◇◇◇◇◇◇◇◇◇◇◇◇◇◇◇◇◇◇◇◇◇◇

Freedom is a beautiful thing, a wondrous gift from a mysterious source, carefully crafted by natural selection for our enjoyment. Once opened, we soon came to learn that the gift of freedom comes with a catch—without a sense of moral responsibility, freedom is dangerous. As a species we are privileged to be free to choose what to believe and how to live, yet we are condemned by our freedom to suffer should we choose unwisely.

Consciousness emerged as a property within living beings. When it did, it would only be a matter of time before freedom would arrive in the hominid brain with its conjoined twin, the moral conscience. Our ancestral line gave birth to an evolving species of self whose sense of freedom was to be balanced by a moral sense. This species of self-consciousness gave rise to language, abstract thought, and advancing knowledge that gave rise to the spread of dynamically complex cultural traditions, social, political and economic systems, and advanced technologies. Perfect freedom would be accompanied by a perfect moral capacity. These gifts have yet to arrive.

In *Freedom Evolves*, Tufts University professor, professor, and cognitive scientist Daniel C. Dennett explains:

> Freedom had to evolve like every other feature of the biosphere, and it continues to evolve today. Freedom is real now, in some happy parts of the world, and those who love it love it wisely, but it is far from inevitable, far from universal.

From the looks of the wave of political uprisings in the Middle East, freedom may be entering a new cultural phase, but it is built into the design that human freedom must be countered by a sense of moral responsibility, or the system could break down. Dennett continues:

> If we understand better how freedom arose, we can do a better job of preserving it for the future, and protecting it from its many natural enemies...we can conceive of better worlds and yearn to get there...Our evolved capacity to reflect gives us—and only us—both the opportunity and the competence to evaluate ends, not just means...This provides, at last, a naturalistic framework within which traditional questions of morality make sense.

With at least a partial freedom to choose behaviors and lifestyles, we evolved at least partial moral responsibility for our actions. We did not set the initial forces of the universe in motion, but we used the progeny of those initial forces to acquire freedom and a moral sense, an inseparable pair of qualities that need maintain a functional balance if we are to achieve a balanced state of health and sustainability.

We sit enthralled as cultural media stealthily shape us into who we are, biasing the way we think, choosing our likes and dislikes for us. At times we sense that we are on a path toward mutually assured decay or destruction unless we can get our act together and make better choices.

Our great challenge will be to mesh varied worlds of values, beliefs, and traditions into a collective will to get global metabolic systems under better relative control. Leaders of an international group working on issues of environmental health and sustainability (see Reid, W. V., et al.) have issued a call to action that describes the five grand challenges of Earth system science:

1. Improve the usefulness of forecasts of future environmental conditions and their consequences for people.

2. Develop, enhance, and integrate observation systems to manage global and regional environmental change.

3. Determine how to anticipate, avoid, and manage disruptive global environmental change.

4. Determine institutional, economic, and behavioral changes to enable effective steps toward global sustainability.

5. Encourage innovation (and mechanisms for evaluation) in technological, policy, and social responses to achieve global sustainability.

The grand challenges read like an integrative care plan that humanity would get if it went to see a planetary medicine doctor. The technological challenges are immense, but the social challenges are far greater. In their paper, *Earth System Science for Global Sustainability,* these environmental scientists write:

Progress in understanding and addressing both global environmental change and sustainable development research requires better integration of social science research.

The Earth system concept refers to the sum total of social, political, economic, and environmental infrastructure and activity.

To keep humanity out of the intensive care unit, it will take more than the integration of social science research with earth system science research—it will take collective will to overcome resistance to cultural change. Overcoming resistance to cultural change is not likely without an adjustment of culture-wide balances between freedom and morality. While cultural change research explores whether there are cultural change tipping points, real life pioneering actions should be able to prove that it is possible to move social, political, and economic dynamics toward more sustainable ways of living, governing, and doing business.

Humanity's narrative on Earth is showing clear signs of a descent into chronic illness. In this narrative, Earth system scientists are not villains who take pleasure in killing the buzz of those who view the Earth as humanity's playground and little else. Earth system scientists realize that they can't change the world by themselves. They need help from governments, cultural and institutional leaders, philanthropists, and, perhaps most importantly, from consumers, who have yet to fully own and manage their collective strength to promote corporate responsibility for health and sustainability.

The Earth system narrative stretches back to the Big Bang. The Bang and deep stretches of time gave rise to genes. Genes gave rise to gene regulation systems, which gave rise to higher forms of intelligence popping with ideas, which gave rise to organized social systems. In this astounding sequence one idea stands out: the possibility of God.

Among all the ideas in human history, none is more potent than the idea that we may have a Maker. The idea of the possibility of God loads human experience with a dichotomy: either we have a Maker, or we don't. The dichotomy forces upon our minds a choice between three basic stances toward the God question:

1. Believe in a Maker (be a believer).

2. Believe in no Maker (be an atheist).

3. Take no position (be an agnostic).

This menu of options raises a clinical question: Could our choice on the God question affect the overall human prospect for health and sustainability? If enough people believe that we have a Maker, what, if anything, would that Maker call us to be and to do? If enough of us believe that we do not have a Maker, or take no position, what, if anything, should we be calling ourselves to be and to do? Are we better off answering a call from our Maker or from ourselves?

Whether you believe or do not believe in a Maker, you beg a key question whose answer currently appears beyond human reach. How and why did something come from nothing? You can believe in a Maker or not, or you can skip the question and move on. But the question never goes away. Neither reason nor science has grounds to fully dismiss the possibility of God.

Imagine that an International Board of Medical Specialties has certified a new medical specialty called planetary medicine. The training program has just graduated its first batch of physicians whose mission is to help the World Health Organization

(WHO) move global cultures toward a more sustainable path to health.

One of these graduates was chosen to lead the task of advising humanity as a whole on what to do with the God idea. Mathea Velby, MD, was either brave or deluded enough to accept such a controversial position, but she earnestly felt called to promote health at cultural levels within the Earth system and she didn't care what other people thought about her decision to take the first position of its kind. Dr. Velby was well schooled in the Big History of the cosmos, the stages of evolution on Earth, and the current nature of humanity's health and sustainability predica-ment. She was chosen because of her thirst to understand and treat the growing tension between cultural values and biological neces-sity that is threatening the functional integrity of living systems.

Her research translated and analyzed the largest collection of structured interviews ever conducted. Over 10,000 interview-ees, representing over 180 distinct cultural groups, were asked a series of questions about God, science, religion, and evolution. Her study concluded that faith and reason must work together to optimize our long-term prospects for health and sustainability.

Dr. V's research found that most people believe we should be free to choose a sacred or secular context for living our lives. Most also agreed that there exists no truly objective basis by which to choose one form of belief over the other. Yet a wide majority believes in the existence of One True God, suggesting that subjec-tive experience can be more persuasive than objective knowledge to the human mind. The health and sustainability consequences of this tendency toward religious belief are not yet clear.

Dr. V knew that her species could not wait for properly designed trials to point the way to wellness. The problems in play are too complex to submit to cause-and-effect research designs. She needed interview data to help construct a granular health narrative for present day humanity.

When the healer's task is to evaluate a complex problem that defies explanation, there is always a need for more information. When the issues are so complex as to extend beyond the reach of reason or science, the patient still turns to the healer for guidance. Dr. V was encouraged by her colleagues at the WHO to view the human species as a whole as her patient, and to use whatever data might be of help in her efforts to design an effective care plan. What is more, they expected her to use her instincts and best judgment when the data were too weak a clinical guide—something frowned upon in most other medical specialties.

Historical data clearly showed that agreeable forms of human coexistence fund social cooperation. Any sustainable Earth system would need much more human social cooperation, much the same way any bodymind needs cooperation from its metabolic systems. So her team focused on what it would take for the sacred and the secular, for theism and atheism, to happily coexist with each other.

Dr. V practiced mindfulness-meditation regularly. She thought that this kind of practice had the potential to become a fundamental component of a new, cross-cultural tradition aimed at health and sustainability. It offered a means by which people of any cultural background might connect with the ground of being in a way that is meaningful to them. It was also a way to achieve at least temporary freedom from their suffering. Her concern was that monotheists seem so wedded to their own ways of being that they view spiritual practices outside of their experience with suspicion. In her interviews, monotheists were less willing to sample new ways of thinking, as if fearful of the consequences from doing so.

She reasoned that theists, atheists, and agnostics must remain free to put their energy into converting people to their beliefs, but that they should be encouraged to explore the meditative practices within their faith traditions, such as contemplative prayer. Functional magnetic resonance imaging research was showing what a difference meditation can make to people who suffer from pain or chronic illness.

Dr. V once compared subcultures opposed to the idea of promoting meditative skills as being like bacteria that are resistant to treatment, only the goal of treatment is not to kill or slow growth, but to heal and promote new growth. Without personal self-regulation, she wondered, how can there be social self-regulation? Without social self-regulation, how can there be global social cooperation?

She knew that any worldview must answer the fundamental ethical question: What are we being called to be and to do? The answer must address both the individuals who comprise the "we" of a given culture, but also the global "we" of all cultures as a whole. Just as the metabolic systems of the individual bodymind seek to maintain a state of functional integrity, so too must the bodymind of humanity. It should be part of every healer's mission to build consensus for health and sustainability as a species-wide goal, and part of every person's mission to become a healer.

Dr. V's parents were cold narcissists who only ever thought about themselves. She was a gifted child though, who fully invested herself in making her parents happy. When she failed at that she sublimated her courage and drive into making the world a friendlier place within her sphere of influence. When she encountered people who said they cared about humanity and the fate of the Earth but upon closer inspection failed to act the part, she would smile and remind herself that behavior change isn't easy. Hearts and minds could be in the right place, but when votes, spending habits, savings habits, and mouse clicks are not, people need more help and encouragement. Humanity, she hypothesized, is in need of pioneering innovations that can help this sizable part of the global population channel its enlightened beliefs into healthier, more sustainable behaviors.

In her new job she was no longer building a theory about health and sustainability—she was in the full swing of medical practice, face to face with a planetary patient as an astoundingly complex whole. She wondered if healers elsewhere in the cosmos were busy attending to planetary health. Her curiosity was so insatiable that she was always desperate for more information. Constructing a planetary health narrative is worth the work, she thought. Best to take one's time and do your level best to understand the patient's problem before jumping to solutions. She often remembered what a favorite teacher had told her: "The first sign of genius is to acknowledge what you don't know."

"The path of evolution," she would say to cheers in her most popular talk, "has gone from creation to genes to consciousness to freedom to now. The only thing missing is the courage to be responsible." After the pause she'd continue, "The key challenge confronting our species is to find a way to balance personal and social freedom with personal and social responsibility." A slow anthem would rise through the loudspeakers as a montage of children from various cultures played on the screen above her. She would conclude that our health and sustainability dilemma was caused by a growing "human responsibility deficit" and that "human freedom must learn to conform itself to the functional integrity of the whole."

She redrew the analogy about our being like frogs in water slowly heating to a boil, to our being like frogs in puddles of polluted water, unaware that hormone-disrupting chemicals are corrupting our systems for reproduction, energy production, cognitive function, immunity, and tumor suppression.

She foretold that our earthly habitat would inevitably force us to curb our freedoms, such as our freedom to turn million-year old raw materials into toxic disposables that litter landscapes and despoil the oceans with the mark of a vandal species.

She warned that human beings are no longer free to ignore the ethical imperative that bears down with equal force on theists and atheists, agnostics and fundamentalists, progressives and conservatives, libertarians and totalitarians, and so on. All are called to seek wisdom, value health, integrate, and aim for a working balance between prosperity and sustainability. The goals of treatment were getting clearer, but for this planetary medicine doctor, the care plan never seemed granular enough. She needed more information.

For cultures to achieve stable and healthy forms and phases of coexistence, she realized that capturing individual hearts and minds would not be enough to change something as complex as a culture, let alone a developing global civilization. She wanted to know more about what is needed for modern cultures to implement healthy change.

A colleague referred her to the work of a social theorist named James Davison Hunter. In *To Change the World*, Davison explains that converting individuals to new ideas, values, beliefs, and behaviors is important, but it is not enough to change a culture whose historical roots run deep and whose embedded institutions and power structures are firmly rooted in the status quo. This is why substantial cultural change—the kind that results in social transformation—usually unfolds over generations, not decades or a few years.

As interconnectedness and open knowledge sharing increase, so in theory will our degrees of freedom for solving global problems that require us to have a more mature relationship with the world and its assets. But unless the resulting vision comes with a plan for influencing the power-wielding elites who lead cultural institutions, it is unlikely to promote major change.

The twentieth century had witnessed more technological advances than all past centuries put together. Now the planet was blanketed with people and their stuff—an accumulation of industrial byproducts (carbon emissions, toxic chemicals, plastics, bent metals, etc.) and unintended consequences (new chronic illness burdens for people and ecosystems) whose impact on the other parts of the planet as a whole were poorly understood but increasingly hazardous and potentially beyond our control.

Hunter observed:

Ideas do have consequences in history, yet not because they are inherently truthful or obviously correct but rather because of the way they are embedded in very powerful institutions, networks, interests, and symbols.

To change a currently dominant set of ideas, even though they are so obviously unsustainable, it is necessary to implant better ideas. But better ideas won't succeed unless they can influence the power-wielding elites. Dr. V's goal was not to receive ebullient congratulations on her presentations. Winning hearts and minds was an objective, but minor in comparison to influencing the power-wielding elites who lead the world's cultural, social, political, and economic institutions.

Hunter noted that such change is usually "initiated by elites who are outside of the centermost positions of prestige" within dominant cultural institutions and networks:

> Wherever innovation begins, it comes as a challenge to the dominant ideas and moral systems defined by the elites who possess the highest levels of symbolic capital. Innovation, in other words, generally moves from elites and the institutions they lead not to the general population but among elites who do not necessarily occupy the highest echelons of prestige. The novelty they represent and offer calls into question the rightness and legitimacy of the established ideas and prac-tices of the culture's leading gatekeepers. The goal of any such innovation is to infiltrate the center and, in time, redefine the leading ideas and practices of the center.

Now she could see that part of her strategy would be to use current social networks to recruit leaders whose positions were not centermost to an institution but close enough to read the pulse and influence thinking with ideas that support global health and sustainability. This component of her strategy would need to be backed by thoughtful methods of communication and access to solid educational resources and references. If multimedia presen-tations were to have a role, they would be designed for the confer-ence room, not the auditorium.

She set out to gather good ideas, new and old, with some bear-ing on humanity's need to come to terms with the importance of functional integration and its implications for human health and the sustainability of living systems. She also realized that she'd need to take an open-minded look at how personal and corporate habits inhibit or promote health and sustainability.

A globalization process was well underway. It had the potential to stabilize or destabilize existing cultures and social structures. It appeared that humanity was becoming a cause of illness within the system as a whole. And if, as she suspected, human know-how had far surpassed its know-why, the prognosis for restoring health would be worse.

In an age when most members of the human species see that the health of ecological systems underwrites its long-term prospects as the dominant presence in the world, its cultures and institutions are plagued by an adaptation defect. This defect does not stem from the way cultures and institutions undermine the health of the living systems, but from their doing so wittingly, knowing that future generations depend on the functional integrity of living systems. The industrialized human presence on Earth has become the chief source of inflammation in the world. Dr. V could see that if humanity failed to suppress the inflammation it was spreading into the Earth's living systems, then people would be freely choosing to become destroyers rather than stewards.

A steward can be a person or an institution or, in the case Dr. V wanted to make, a global civilization that is entrusted to care for a valuable resource that it does not own. In middle schools and high schools she would give a presentation that got things started this way: "Does humanity own the Earth? Is the Earth a valuable resource? Are we good stewards of the Earth? How can we become better stewards of the Earth?" The vociferous No-Yes-No response got the adrenalin going for answers to her question. After two hours the kids were still fully engaged and didn't want the session to end. The teachers would then introduce ways of tying health and sustainability concerns into their curricula using tools supplied by Dr. V's team.

Notice that this planetary medicine doctor had no evidence-based answers on how to proceed; she had to induce her way to explanatory power and a care plan that made sense based on what power she had to explain an extraordinarily complex problem. To build a narrative for our species, she wanted access to all the information she could get her hands on. She did not artificially restrict the information gathering process. If she was to get serious about doing what it takes to promote functional integrity at multiple levels within her spheres of influence, then she would need to dig deep within the narrative to find sustainable ways to reconcile our conflicting beliefs and ideologies, and then sweep away the obstacles hiding in the corridors of power.

She knew that a division between science and religion exists within many subcultures around the world. The toughest divisions to overcome are often those that exist between particular faith traditions within a given religion, or between denominations within a faith tradition. She wondered if an integrative problem-solving approach had been taken to the issue of creating a more functional level of integration among differing Christian beliefs. She also wanted a way to define what differentiates healthy from unhealthy Christian forms of belief and practice.

In his last major work, *Religion within the Limits of Reason Alone,* German philosopher Immanuel Kant (1724–1804) wrote, "If it provides for us a unified whole of systematically ordered activities, our acts constitute in general a *service* of God." This idea deeply resonated with Dr. V. To Kant, a healthy living system is a unified whole of activities, systematically ordered. She felt that promoting health and order within living systems would, for most religious believers, be viewed as a fitting response to their Maker.

Kant's was not a clinical philosophy. He didn't approach the subjects of faith and reason from a health angle. He sought to provide a logical foundation for religious belief because supernatural revelations weren't trustworthy ways to describe reality. They still aren't, though that doesn't mean they are without value.

Kant could justify the rituals of prayer, evangelism, baptism, and communion— religious traditions derived from revelations—only when their intention was to further the moral good. He despised hypocrisy in all of its forms, but especially in faith traditions when he sensed that revelations were being used to mislead the faithful. In this way he drew the distinction between healthy (good) religion and unhealthy (bad) religion.

Good religion inspires its adherents to love the good, to do the right thing, and keep aiming higher for a more fitting response to a Maker. Good religion can adopt supernatural revelations, but it refuses to toss a scientific understanding of reality out the window. Good religion can certainly inspire human beings to become better stewards of the functional integrity of living systems. Dr. V saw that good religion would have a positive role to play in the clinical philosophy she was building.

Whether or not beliefs advocated by good religion describe fundamental truths about reality, she figured, the beliefs are valuable to us because of their inspirational and health-promoting power. We need health-promoting power for a Maker's creation to flourish on our watch. Good religion would seem to be a fitting response to any Maker in any universe.

Bad religion, on the other hand, amplifies the divisions that separate different groups and throws obstacles in front of cultural efforts to promote the health and functional integrity of social systems. This is in part because the centermost power-wielders in bad religious traditions are highly resistant to change from the outside.

In bad religion, defending the interests of the leaders in power is more important than promoting the functional integration of all the Maker's people. The result might be a fatwa that calls for the death of a man for committing the sin of free speech, or a Papal inquisition that authorizes the activities of anti-heretic squads.

It is not the fatwa or the Papal encyclical itself that is good or bad; it is the purpose and substance of it, and what it prompts believers to do in the name of God. Religion is bad when its moral codes are dexterously used to support tyranny, self-aggrandizement, or terror in the name of God. Kant worried that leaders within various historical religious traditions sought to "manage to their own advantage the Invisible Power which presides over the destiny of men," and that they would use supernatural revelations as a management tool for their own benefit.

Kant chastised spiritual guides who would lead their flocks to believe that mere profession of faith could suffice as genuine service to our Maker, especially if such faith emphasizes dogmatic rules and rituals over the cultivation of virtuous conduct in all of one's affairs. Perhaps we are saved by God's grace, but that is no excuse to neglect what your Maker is calling us to be and to do.

Kant came to the subject of Christian belief from a philosophical point of view. His message was a call to serve God by focusing on the essence of what Jesus taught by his example. In Kant's opinion, a religious denomination is capable of promoting religious beliefs and practices that are good or bad. Multiple denominations or different shades of belief are not the problem; flock manipulation by religious leadership defending their power interests is the problem. That was not what Jesus was about. If the Church is to be about the example of Jesus, then what, specifically, should the Church be about?

A friend of Dr. V's recommended the book *Your Church Is Too Small*, by John Armstrong, who takes the position that the time has come for the main branches of Christianity (Protestant, Catholic, and Eastern Orthodox) to unite around their most sacred shared belief: that the human path should be lit and inspired by the teachings of Jesus.

Armstrong's initial call for *post-denominationalism* drew intense heat. Flame-throwing critics reacted by defending the superiority of their denominations over the rest. Any new idea can threaten to loosen some leader's grip on earthly power. When that leader is a Christian, claws may come out in the name of Jesus.

Armstrong notes that the original purpose of Christian religious rules and rituals was to keep believers focused on the main beam that would hold up the central mission of the church: to remain true to what God calls us to be and to do by reference to the life, death, and resurrection of Jesus.

The splintering of the Church into dozens of new denominations with their own rules and rituals is not the issue, thought Dr. V. The issue is how this tempts church organizers to drift away from the central mission of Christianity. Deviating from the central mission invites members of the larger community of Christians to engage in the "us versus them" style of thinking that keeps culture wars up and running as obstacles to health and sustainability.

Diversity among Christian churches is not the problem. The problem is that for any new doctrines relating to the central mission of Christian practice, some will find new ways to serve the Lord, and others will find new ways to serve themselves in the name of the Lord.

The net effect of tacking a growing variety of rules and rituals onto the main mission of the church has been a loss of Christian coherence over time. Because this erodes the ecumenical spirit that seeks unity and friendly relations among the Christian churches of the world, Armstrong sounds a call for *missional-ecumenism*, a movement that supports the reformation of Christianity as a whole by recalibrating it to a renewed commitment to its central mission: love of God and one another.

Dr. V wanted to draw attention to this growing spirit of togetherness about the mission of the main branches of Christianity in the world. Sharing renewed focus on their main missions could build bridges of friendship, trust, and collaboration among members of all the world's religions, provided their leaders are motivated to find common moral and spiritual ground. Missional-ecumenism would represent a functional new dynamic in efforts to orient religious cultures toward the requirements of health and sustainability.

Part of meeting the grand challenges of Earth system sustainability will involve new collaborations among the world's religious traditions. A world organized around principles of health and wellness would be a fitting way to serve any Maker of any universe, and a wise path for the species to take in any event, Maker or not.

As Dr. V gained a deeper understanding of what the developing world bodymind needed from humanity, bits and pieces of a care plan started coming into view. This care plan in formation was definitely a product of an integrative clinical mind-set that took applied systems biology perspective to the cultural change problems at hand. That is, Dr. V sensed that cultures have metabolic interactions of their own that point our species toward social wellness or social ills. The physiology of health and sustainability would require a more responsible use of human freedom to create stabilizing forms of functional integration within and between human cultures.

Though the path to health and sustainability remains unclear, we can see that our species needs to make tracks toward the functional integration of religious traditions. Freedom of religion stands for freedom to believe whatever you want to believe. As a result, we find good religions focused on what God requires of us, and bad religions focused on what we require of God. Good religious belief cannot be forced; it must be freely chosen. With religious freedom comes the responsibility to submit to the ideals and requirements of something greater than our selves.

Ultimately, no health paradigm can be considered whole that fails to relate itself to the fundamental context for all being. All forms of wisdom in our universe are products of complex interacting systems whose origins reach back to a mysterious source.

The Source of All Wisdom

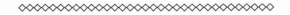

When you process information at a conscious level, you interpret it, give it meaning, decide whether it matters to you, and then determine what, if anything, you should do in response to it. How you respond depends on things you have already learned. What you learn depends on what is taught, how it's taught, how closely you pay attention, and how much you are moved to care. Over time, knowledge and values form the beliefs that become your personal view of the world. Dr. V understood that there was a complex interplay between culture of origin and the development of personal views of the world. These world-views often develop in a haphazard way, with little guidance as to what constitutes wisdom or virtue.

She saw at least three control points for wisdom self-regulation in the Earth system: interactions between leaders of cultural institutions, interactions between parents and children, and inter-actions between the environment and people going through the adolescent-to-young adult transition.

So much of what happens during the preschool years determines whether the developing self will approach life from a stance of fear or trust. The adolescent transition into adulthood is the crucible of character development, a blazing furnace of emotion that forges circuits that can influence lifelong behaviors.

So Dr. Velby and her planetary medicine team got busy on a proposal to create an institution of their own, called the One Bodymind Institute-World Action Network. Known affectionately as OBI-WAN, the institute's mission was to build a global social network to promote education and cultural change aimed at the long-term health and sustainability of humanity and the Earth's living systems. They would launch it with a major initiative called The Wisdom Project.

Their idea was to trace the course of wisdom—and its associated cardinal virtues of prudence, justice, temperance, and courage—from infancy through adulthood, looking for educational opportunities that might benefit parents and teachers from any culture of origin.

Resistance came from all directions, most of it concerned that the Project was an attempt to position Western philosophy and Christianity as the judge and jury for what counts as wisdom and virtue for the species.

There was no denying that the concept of tying wisdom to these cardinal virtues traced back to Plato (423-347 BC), and that it became a linchpin of Catholic moral thinking from Ambrose (337-397) and Augustine (354-430) to Aquinas (1225-1274) and Pascal (1623-1662). The Institute's multicultural Board of Advisors had approved the project aware of this concern, but they did not anticipate the firestorm of criticism on the social networks, let a lone the staged protests outside their facility in Geneva.

Of course other wisdom traditions would be actively worked into the process of assembling a cultural framework for parenting and education based on practical wisdom and virtue.

Every effort would be made to incorporate not the mere findings of science related to parenting, education, and character development, but the most meaningful interpretations of scientific findings—bearing in mind that wisdom is tempered by something much like the four cardinal virtues, though Eastern cultural wisdom and mystic wisdom traditions would have much more to add to the discussion.

The resistance movement fizzled out once respected religious, scientific, and social leaders from leading institutions in dozens of countries signed on for a two-year commitment to interviews and task force work aimed at a World Charter for Cultural Wisdom. The aim of the Charter would be to gather the most practical wisdom from science, religion, and specific cultural traditions that relates to the shaping of the personal worldviews and character needed to advance our species toward a more stable platform for health and sustainability.

The OBI-WAN team recovered from their early misstep by securing participation from 100 culturally diverse institutional leaders. Press coverage all but vanished after the team and their panel of participants dove into action. When they re-emerged fifteen months later, they had a 2,000-page document for academics and professionals, and a condensed version for the lay public.

Much of the Wisdom Project's report outlined the fundamental necessities of maternal and child health, proposing novel approaches to getting these needs met in underprivileged countries, including the creation of a world coalition of non-governmental organizations whose missions relate to child health.

There was total consensus around the idea that culture is a product of worldviews and that worldviews form over time as social forces shape the more primitive biological forces that underlie human behavior. As you pass through childhood, the core aspects of your self are jostling around, vying for the best seats in your *unconscious* mind. In most people, the neural circuits of emotion determine behavioral responses before rational capacities have had time to react. This process can lead to a host of anxiety-driven addictive behaviors that become increasingly hard to control when the brain's reward pathways grow used to expecting each next time to feel better than the last time. Addictive behaviors can be ruinous to human health and sustainability.

Since our conscious minds use various filters to try to make sense of and control the urges and impulsive reactions that can run us toward ruin, freedom from addiction and anxiety seems to require reasonably well-developed self-regulation skills. Near the top of any list of care plan components for childrearing and education humanity was the recommendation that children from all cultures get the chance to experience the benefits of mindfulness by learning self-regulation skills. These skills could derive from traditions within the family's culture of origin, or from a different cultural tradition. The important thing was to transfer such skills to as many children as possible before adolescence so the developing self can enter adolescence and the transition to young adulthood with a skill set that promotes an ability to maintain some semblance of physical and emotional balance.

The authors were concerned that as our beliefs become more or less settled in our minds, they fall into patterns that identify us with the communities and cultural traditions that most influenced our maturation process. They gave an example of what a difference prevailing culture can make.

If you live in Afghanistan under the rule of the Taliban, distributing an essay on women's rights could earn you twenty years in jail. If you live in the United States, filing a lawsuit asserting a woman's right to equal pay for equal work could result in a Supreme Court precedent that makes it illegal for corporations to base pay on gender. Finding a shared cross-cultural sense of purpose is no easy task when similar ideals and motivations mean overtly different things from one culture to another.

What societies do with their cases of criminal and civil injustice depends on what their dominant culture teaches and on what citizens and their leaders have learned to believe, commit to practice, and translate into custom or law.

Some people pray; some do not. Some who pray do so while kneeling on a bench, facing a cross. Others kneel with their heads to the floor, facing Mecca. Some can hear a wood thrush sing and collapse into the ocean of being. These are all ways of connecting to something higher than ourselves, of feeling inspired to be and to do something more than sit around all day eating fake food and living empty lives. The different customs and rituals are products of cultures that exist on a spectrum between open and tolerant to closed and intolerant.

The Report also took the position that the ability of cultural variations to peacefully coexist side-by-side depends on the openness of educational institutions and their ability to tolerate different systems of belief and ways of being. On the whole, intolerance breeds intolerance, and intolerance reduces our capacity for social cooperation. Since social cooperation is a functional requirement of health and sustainability, the authors recommended that both parents and educators around the world take a closer look at the juggernaut known as *Khan Academy*, a radically open and personalized system for learning that, in the home, supports knowledge transfer and, in the classroom, makes tolerance and cooperation a natural part of the educational process.

"One of the great challenges for world cultures in the twenty-first century," they wrote, "will be achieving progressively higher forms of functional integration based on education and social cooperation." The authors cited Khan Academy as an emergent phenomenon that is changing the culture of education, and that has great potential for supporting social evolution toward health and sustainability. "The Earth system," they wrote, "is poised to witness another major transition in the evolution of social systems, one in which the now dominant species, *Homo sapiens*, achieves a transformative level of social cooperation."

In *The Principles of Social Evolution*, Andrew F. G. Bourke, professor of evolutionary biology at the University of East Anglia, describes the evolution of social systems on Earth as a series of six major transitions. The last of these transitions produced what ecologists call *interspecific mutualisms*—the patterns and processes by which species come to depend on each other. Each transition along the way recapitulates a basic pattern and process. Bourke describes it this way:

> The major transitions view helps explain the increase in the complexity of living things over evolutionary time. It does this in two ways. One arises simply because a nested hierarchy is necessarily more complex than each of its lower-level constituents. The other comes about because each major transition creates conditions for the evolution of mechanisms for

excluding would-be exploiters and for reducing internal conflict, [mechanisms] which themselves add to the overall complexity of the new level. If the selfish interests of the formerly independent units cannot be sufficiently subordinated to the collective interest of the higher-level entity, such an entity will be unstable and the transition to a new level [of socially stable complexity] will fail.

The chapter of human history that we're living in this century thus contains an important pivot point in the evolutionary plot line. Can we integrate diverse cultural systems in a way that preserves their diversity while enhancing their ability to function in healthy and sustainable ways?

In the recent history of human culture, five mechanisms that facilitate higher-order functional integration are worth noting:

1. Promoting specialized work and trade.

2. Balancing economic development with natural resource management.

3. Leveraging human cognitive surplus and the wisdom of the crowd.

4. Rewarding innovation and meaningful new ideas.

5. Empowering ordinary people with extraordinary technologies.

In *The Rational Optimist*, Matt Ridley makes the case for specialization and trade as forces that naturally move people in the direction of happiness and a standard of living characterized by more free time. In a world of specialists offering quality products, services, and skills, people don't have to spend all of their time getting their needs for food, shelter, and conveniences met by personally learning the necessary techniques and doing the work themselves.

Self-sufficiency is an admirable trait, worthy of emulation for many reasons, but specialists trading products and skills with each other is a way of creating value that has the benefit of creating more free time for people—a marker of a better standard of living.

Trade began as a local phenomenon in the distant past. By ten thousand years ago, a typical Sumerian market might have offered grains, fish, meat, pelts, cloth, twine, tools, metals, beads, pottery, and lottery tickets.

The beauty of the system was that trade had a way of turning enemies into trade partners. Instead of fighting each other over natural resources such as minerals and grazing grounds, people could trade their goods or skills for other assets that were harder to come by, freeing up more time for them to enjoy life and become productive in new ways—such as, say, attending more closely to the intellectual and emotional lives of their children.

It didn't take long for trade to go regional. Once shipping became possible, trade went global. More recently, international free trade has put intense pressure on jobs in developed parts of the world. But the movement of jobs to less-developed parts of world is what helps poor countries elevate the standard of living in ways that can lift families out of poverty. One country's pinch point is another country's path to prosperity.

But prosperity always comes at some kind of cost. With the expansion of foreign trade opportunities, we accelerate our consumption of the Earth's natural assets because more people find their way into jobs that lead them a step closer to more modern ways of consuming natural resources. Oxford economist Paul Collier, former director of the Development Research Group at the

World Bank, lays out the intricacies of natural asset management in his book *The Plundered Planet*.

Natural assets include nonrenewable subsoil assets such as oil and minerals, as well as renewable assets such as food crops. The job of finding subsoil assets like oil, minerals, and precious metals is costly and financially risky. Governments and private firms dance around who's going to pay how much for absorbing this risk. Once they are located, the job of extracting these assets carries some risk as well. When things go wrong, as they did with the *Deepwater Horizon* rig in the Gulf of Mexico, the blame game begins.

The problem that environmentalists have with economic globalization is the rate at which global consumption is depleting nonrenewable assets, and the way governments and private firms discount the side effects of pollution and habitat loss. At the same time, those working to end poverty and raise the standard of living for the bottom billion will accept certain forms of depletion or damage to the environment in order to achieve their social, economic, and humanitarian goals.

Food crops are renewable assets but supply is not meeting global demand for food. One answer to this problem, genetic modification (GM), is another hot button. Corporate agribusiness stepped up to the challenge of feeding the world's hungry—and then got pilloried by the green movement for creating "Frankenfoods." The green movement counters by asserting the *precautionary principle* as the way to manage risks to human health and the functional integrity of living systems. If we sacrifice a precautionary approach on the altar of economic development, they say, we are more likely to suffer the *law of unintended consequences*.

An example of an unintended consequence of a GM food would be the effects that can follow the use of Roundup Ready seed crops. Roundup is an herbicide (glyphosate) made by the corporation Monsanto. Roundup concentrates in soil and water runoff, and can disrupt vertebrate reproductive hormonal pathways, being somewhat more toxic to fish and amphibians. The Environmental Protection Agency (EPA) classifies it as slightly toxic to people, which means harmful if swallowed, inhaled, or absorbed through the skin.

GM crops engineered to be Roundup Ready are primarily soybeans and corn, though versions for alfalfa, beets, canola, cotton, and wheat are being developed. Weeds that have become resistant to Roundup are designated superweeds. Cotton farmers in the Southeastern United States are increasingly losing their crops to a Roundup-resistant plant called pigweed.

Some studies show that Roundup Ready wheat is more susceptible to head blight caused by a fungus called *fusarium*. This fungus makes a toxin called DON (short for deoxynivalenol), which has been shown to cause intestinal permeability in human intestinal cells. Should this toxin survive on processed wheat products and piggyback into the guts of people who are unaware of their gluten intolerance, the result would be a rise in medically unexplained and potentially disabling illness.

What, then, could possibly justify the use of Roundup Ready crops? There are some important benefits touted by Monsanto and agriculturalists. They include weed control and the multiple advantages of reducing the need for tillage as a weed-control strategy. Tillage reduces surface-layer soil nutritional content, promotes soil erosion, and increases toxic fertilizer and pesticide runoff. Reducing tillage reduces these risks and can increase the farmer's profit margin by reducing manual labor costs. Though it isn't yet clear whether Roundup Ready crops generate higher yields, the use of Roundup has some merit.

Yet we know very little about the safety and biodiversity effects produced when we engineer genes and transfer them into crop species. The Union of Concerned Scientists contends that human-engineered and transferred genes, or *transgenes*, will have effects that are far more complex than we can know or predict. We did not anticipate, for example, that cross-pollination would result in *gene drift*—a process by which native species of plant become contaminated with transgenes, perhaps speeding the development of herbicide resistant superweeds.

A group called ETC tracks activities that affect food safety and crop biodiversity. They warn that giant agrochemical companies are engaged in a widespread patent grab that could give them eventual control over much of the world's plant biomass. They can do this by trading royalty-free seeds in return for lax regulatory constraints—ideal conditions for inducing farmers to become dependent on genetically engineered crops.

Dr. Vandana Shiva's research demonstrates that organic farming methods can produce up to five times as much food per acre as farming that uses industrial chemicals and transgenes to increase yields of single species crops. Her Navdanya Biodiversity Farm in India stockpiles seeds instead of patents. She has over 1,500 seed varieties that she grows under varied stress conditions to produce resistance to environmental stress the way nature does—natural selection of genes and epigenetic modifications that enhance the ability of a species to adapt to changes in its environment. Human micromanagement of the plant biomass natural selection process has the markings of a modern day Pandora's box. As well-intentioned,

patent-driven industrial opportunities trump precautionary concerns for the umpteenth time, we may encounter gene spills whose
consequences cannot be undone.

The question of whether or not to use Roundup Ready
GM crops symbolizes the complexity of our health and sustainability problem. "If crops don't adapt to climate change,
neither will agriculture, and neither will we," noted Cary
Fowler, Executive Director of the Global Crop Diversity Trust
at a 2009 TED conference. Renee Cho of the Earth Institute
at Columbia University reported, "For every one degree
Centigrade rise above optimum growing temperatures, farmers will likely experience a ten percent decline in their yields."
The pressure on farmers to increase yields is enormous. Cho
points out that "with growing population expected to hit nine
billion by 2050, eighty million more people will need to be
fed each year."

We can either ignore the precautionary principle and the law
of unintended consequences, or we can let millions of people go
hungry. Western societies agonize over the toxicity question, but
as a government official from an African country once put it, "You
Westerners are within your rights to discuss the pros and cons of
genetically modified crops, but in the meantime, can we eat?"

Collier draws an important distinction between the concept of
environmental conservation (no net loss) and that of environmental stewardship (planned gains and losses). None of the Earth's
natural assets can be considered permanently sustainable if they
can either be extracted all the way down to zero, or to a point
where zero additional extraction can be achieved. Humanity is
reaching the place in its history where better stewardship of living systems is imperative. Difficult choices are inescapable.

The OBI-WAN Wisdom Project tackled this issue as well. Dr. V wrote, "It seems highly unlikely that we'll be able pull the bottom billion up to a decent standard of living without the help of new methods to increase crop yields, and without extracting nonrenewable natural assets at an increased rate for several decades. In addition," she added, "the volatility of future geopolitical power struggles may depend in part on what the developed world does to help the bottom billion satisfy their basic human needs for food, shelter, work, meaning, and dignity. Wise and virtuous parenting and education does little good for children who are hungry and sick all the time. Being born luckier than most of the world's billions, the well off are also born more obligated."

As global populations become more closely connected, geopolitical strategy will increasingly entail winning hearts and minds online. Dr. V wrote, "There are over a billion hearts and minds that won't be won unless we can keep their stomachs filled. For a challenge this big, cultural change through new ideas able to penetrate the centermost corridors of power needs to join the winning of hearts and minds."

The sustainability issue, then, from a health and wellness standpoint, is not about protecting the environment at *all* costs, nor is it about looking the other way as global developers and traders plunder the environment. The middle road is to functionally integrate an ethic of environmental and cultural stewardship with a vision of human flourishing that remains consistent with long-term health and sustainability goals.

Development is not the enemy. Environmental protection is not a curse. Plunder and apathy are the enemies. Unintended consequences are the curse. Corruption, negligence, and misplaced priorities are ushering us into an age of toxic burdens and genetic misadventures that will affect the privileged and underprivileged in near equal measure.

It is often a new synthesis of ideas, a stronger problem-solving paradigm that pulls hearts and minds to a cause. In the case of integrative problem solving of the medical sort, actual solutions depend on a realistic understanding of a patient's systems biology. Wherever a care plan requires cultural change, actual solutions will depend on a realistic understanding both of systems biology *and* of specific social institutions and their change dynamics. Sometimes, however, cultures change on their own.

Driven by cost control, technology, and new labor trends, many institutions and industries are changing on their own. In *A Whole New Mind*, Daniel Pink draws a distinction between the Information Age (the 1990s to the present) and the Conceptual Age (now and going forward). The combination of material abundance, the expansion of Asian labor markets, and the computerized automation of work have changed the nature of what it means to be a knowledge worker in the new world economy.

The transition from managing information to creating meaningful new ideas is causing a jobs crisis in the Western world, but in every crisis there is opportunity. Pink argues that the labor markets of the world as a whole are shifting to reward workers with a new set of aptitudes, based on a shortage of people with talents for right-brained creativity and synthesis as opposed to left-brained logic and analysis.

The greatest rewards will go to employees or self-employed consultants who help create products or services that demonstrate a knack for the most prized aptitudes of the Conceptual Age: the abilities to synthesize new ideas in meaningful ways, to design increasingly practical and artful solutions to various problems, and to develop compelling storylines that evoke empathy and encourage play and participation.

In *The Great Reset*, economist Richard Florida predicts a somewhat different change in the recovering American economy that will rewrite the rules for success in the decades to come:

> Two sets of skills matter more now: *analytical* skills, such as pattern recognition and problem solving, and *social intelligence* skills, such as the situational sensitivity and persuasiveness required for team building and mobilization.

Plan on having a good ability to synthesize new ideas and solve problems using both the left and the right sides of your brain, realizing that these are the skills needed by people being put to work on the complex issues that will challenge us for decades to come.

Cultural observer Clay Shirky observes that free time plus motive, plus means, plus opportunity, equals surplus of practical intelligence looking for something meaningful to do—a vast reservoir of knowledge and experience that lies dormant in the minds of the Web-enabled. This valuable resource is always out there, waiting to be put to use for a good cause.

In *Cognitive Surplus*, Shirky discusses the potential for social networking websites to change the way people approach health and self-care:

> These sites must aggregate user data in ways that offer [users] a sense of membership and shared effort. For these users, participation feels like a shift from a cultural norm where medical professionals hoard information and hide it from patients—to a norm of sharing in which everyone benefits.

At *onebodymind.com* we're building a community around principles of health and wellness, where laypeople and professionals come to learn, create, and share ideas for leading healthier lives. We're honored to be in a position to help organize cognitive surplus for the sake of human health and sustainable stewardship of the Earth.

Dr. V's team gained mostly positive recognition for their accomplishments with the Wisdom Project. They received funding from thousands of contributors around the world. Corporations wanted to be on the right side of the health and sustainability issue. Together they donated over seventy million dollars to OBI-WAN. Donations comprised of dollar bills and handwritten thank you cards came from elementary school classes around the world, many of which had integrated Khan Academy and other programs into their method of teaching.

With all this support, The Wisdom Project moved into its next phase: new technologies to empower average citizens in their efforts to promote wisdom, virtue, health, and sustainable forms of resource stewardship. The team was especially interested in using social networks to recruit volunteers to healthy causes. There was a particular interest in what might be done to empower citizens to stem corruption, intolerance, and abuse. They wanted an early detection system to help stop such behavior in its tracks, before extreme intolerance could lead to the dehumanization and killing of innocent people. Such a system could help us create a world without genocide,

A senior member of Dr. V's team had been a police commissioner. He said they would need a surveillance mechanism that could outmaneuver the forces of corruption. Dr. V asked, "What would such a mechanism look like?"

An office intern said, "It would look like this," holding her cell phone above her head. "All you need are people with smart phones drawn to where the action is." She had the group pull out their smart phones, pull up their browsers, and search "ushahidi."

The word *ushahidi* is Swahili for "testimony" or "witness." It is also the name of an organization that came into being during the post-election violence in Kenya in 2008. At *ushahidi.com*, anyone with a smart phone can post photos, video, or texts, and anyone with an Internet-enabled computer can submit detailed reports concerning crisis-related happenings anywhere in the world. Their open-source software uses crowd-sourcing algorithms to track, filter, and map user posts concerning outbreaks of violence, natural disasters, the spread of epidemic infections, election fraud, and other events that warrant rapid communication and response.

The result thus far is something like a rapid early-detection response for noxious social or biological developments as they occur, wherever smart phones, computers, and Web connectivity are present.

Smart phone images and texts brought the Kenyan ballot fraud and violence to a fairly abrupt halt. Fraudulent electioneers realized that they were losing their carefully guarded reputations by the minute. Unlike words on paper, words and images posted by organized groups of individuals in real time have a deterrent effect on perpetrators who don't want to get on the wrong side of the crowd.

Early detection makes a difference when it can trigger an effective adaptive or regulatory response. A new idea sprang to life in Kenya in 2008, and a new type of civilian neighborhood watch program came into being. Now *ushahidi.com* is a resource for countering corruption, increasing transparency, mapping responses, and mobilizing relief efforts in real time.

When the earthquake-tsunami struck East Japan on March 11, 2011, a team of volunteers launched *sinsai.info* within four hours of the quake. Using the *ushahidi* platform, they collected over nine thousand reports in the first month and over one million page views. Heavy users included the Japanese government, Google, and Yahoo.

That high use rate reflected the penetration rate of Facebook and Twitter in Japan. Their reach would have been even higher if not for the power outages and extensive infrastructure damage caused by the tsunami. Moderators for *sinsai.info* were able to incorporate hash-tagged tweets into their summary reports, giving them a fine-grained detail not available through other sources. Thus social networks play a role in the success of an early detection and surveillance platform like *ushahidi's*, whose dynamic reflects a cultural immune system at work, finding new ways to help promote wellness and prevent social ills.

Then a secretary mentioned actor George Clooney's privately funded Sentinel Satellite Project as another example of the spontaneous generation of immune-like surveillance systems promoting social responsibility. Installed to monitor and detect destabilizing movements in trouble spots along the border between northern and southern Sudan, satellite images were ready to be broadcast to world media sources within a day or two as a way to stop outbreaks of violence before they happened.

The effectiveness of this methodology is uncertain, but even the threat of broadcasting images may already have acted as a deterrent, as such images would strip the culprits of plausible deniability for their crimes.

The Sentinel Satellite project is a private-sector innovation in preventive crisis diplomacy. It has also been described as a kind of anti-genocide paparazzi—a sublime redirection of the camera's eye away from *schadenfreude* (pleasure in seeing the pain of others) to its moral opposite: the prevention of pain and suffering. These are innovations that can help nudge interdependent societies toward less corruption and violence and greater stability.

Dr. V thanked the staff for their contributions and said to the group, "Efforts like these are inspiring, yet they leave begging a deeper clinical question about root causes. How is our species to deal with its intercultural differences and hatreds?"

A ripe old social anthropology professor suggested that the team might find insight in something called *inclusive fitness theory*. He supplied some background for their conversation and a detailed discussion commenced.

First proposed by evolutionary biologist W. D. Hamilton (1936–2000) in 1964, the most succinct summary of inclusive fitness theory is known as *Hamilton's Rule*, which states that the inclusive fitness of an organism is the sum of how many offspring it co-produces plus the number of offspring it can add to the species by supporting other members of the species.

In a more human context, broadened beyond offspring counts to quality of life, inclusive fitness is the sum of an individual's overall productivity and quality of life during a lifetime, plus the overall productivity and quality of the life of all members of the species within the individual's sphere of influence over time. Analyzing human psychology and behavior, Hamilton identified four basic types of social actions that influence an individual's inclusive fitness level:

- Cooperation: We both win.

- Altruism: I lose so you can win.

- Selfishness: I win, but you lose.

- Spite: We both lose.

Hamilton proposed that natural selection perpetuates altruism, because the offspring of the altruist are more likely to share genes that predispose to selfless behavior. He also thought that altruists may better sense altruistic behaviors in others and reward such tendencies helping to spread the genes that promote altruism.

In *The Selfish Gene*, evolutionary biologist Richard Dawkins countered that natural selection might favor those who mimic altruistic behavior without incurring the costs of caring for others, making them more competitive in the game of survival of the fittest. Dawkins used Hamilton's work as a springboard for his own gene's-eye view of evolution, which holds that evolution has become a contest in which genes compete for their own survival based on the survival advantages they confer to their vehicle organisms.

Naturally, there are other points of view about what drives evolution, but many of the pieces come together when evolution is viewed as a series of major social transitions. In their 1995 work, *The Major Transitions in Evolution*, evolutionary biologist John Maynard Smith and biochemist Eörs Szathmáry outlined the major transitions for a professional audience. Their lay translation, *The Origins of Life*, appeared in 1999.

In *The Principles of Social Evolution*, Bourke condenses the Smith-Szathmáry list of major transitions from eight down to six for the sake of simplicity. His version of the major social evolutionary transitions can be described as follows, with each stage exhibiting a climb to a more complex but stable form of social cooperation:

1. Self-replicating genes find shelter enclosed within the first cell membranes. These cell-enclosed genes, or *prokaryotes*, appear some 3.8 billion years ago.

2. Prokaryotes fuse, forming larger cells called *eukaryotes*, known for their acquisition of mitochondria, the generation of a nucleus and cytoskeleton, and the formation of specialized organelles for protein assembly and repair. These cells appear some two billion years ago.

3. Eukaryotes acquire the ability to reproduce by combining the genes of one cell with the genes of another, roughly 1.6 billion years ago. This *sexual form of reproduction* sets a more rapid pace of change for living systems.

4. Sexually reproducing eukaryotes develop into *simple multicelled organisms*, such as red algae and flagellates, some five hundred million years ago.

5. *Complex multi-celled organisms* divide among their cell types the labor required to raise healthy offspring. They *form within-species systems for social cooperation*. This behavior appeared roughly five hundred million years ago.

6. *Mutually dependent forms of social cooperation between species* appear as early as four hundred million years ago.

Bourke proposes that each transition moves through a cycle of stages:

1. Social group formation

2. Social group maintenance

3. Social group transformation

One can imagine that a textbook of the principles of planetary medicine would draw a clear link between social cooperation and the health and sustainability of living systems, whatever may be the current stage in the unfolding series of social evolutionary transitions.

The Earth system has given rise to a dominant animal whose within-species systems for social cooperation are no longer instinctive. This is because the human genome gave rise to free will and a moral sense, and these have introduced such wide variations in social values and behaviors that the species struggles with its own group maintenance—let alone the maintenance of cooperation with other species. In this way, humanity appears to be devolving toward a state less capable of recognizing or acting upon the patterns and processes of interdependence between species.

"So," went Dr. V, "if the evolution of living systems on Earth remains true to the pattern it has shown across six major transitions over almost four billion years, then humanity needs to smell the coffee of social cooperation. The question, from the standpoint of our integrative mind-set, is how?"

The team was already exploring ways to remove the wedge separating good religion from good science, having reached consensus after heated debate on the definition of "good" so they could agree on what it meant to sort good from bad forms religious and scientific practice. It is faith and science put to a deceitful purpose that threatens the health and happiness of the innocent being misled. In all cultures lies and deceit can ruin prospects for social cooperation by leaving wounds that ache for generations. They began a series of discussions on how particular worldviews might affect our chances for achieving a healthier, more sustainable relationship to each other and the world.

They noted that human faith and reason had now become just as much a part of the whole as energy and mass. If physics and metaphysics are inseparable in human experience, they wondered, then why do people get uneasy with the idea of faith and reason working together toward the same end of health and sustainability? We are wiser when good faith and good science are working together, dumber when they're split, and dumber still when they denigrate each other. From a clinical standpoint, when wisdom held by faith is disconnected from wisdom held by reason, we lose degrees of freedom for solving our health and sustainability problems. This disconnection is pathological.

Our minds fuse objective and subjective aspects of reality into an indivisible experiential whole. If we try to reduce this fused whole into its component parts, we may grasp insights about those parts, but we have taken our focus off the function of the whole. From a clinical standpoint, it is the organism as a whole whose health is sought.

Splitting faith away from reason yields the school of thought known as scientific naturalism, sometimes called evolutionary naturalism, which holds that nature is all there is and that it has no discernable purpose. If nature has no purpose, then humanity has no purpose. This way of thinking forces people to try and reconcile their yearning for meaning and purpose in life with the assertion that nature, life, and being human have no purpose. If our goal is health and sustainability, then the dead-end existentialist worldview of evolutionary naturalism is medically inadvisable.

The weak theological counter to scientific naturalism is that it rests on a shaky assumption: the idea that since nature can appear to have no discernable purpose, it must be true.

The strong theological counter to scientific naturalism is this: given the course of the major evolutionary transitions thus far within the Earth system—and the new wrinkle created by genes losing control to human free will and thus becoming highly dependent on the human moral sense in the process—nature does indeed appear to have a purpose, and that is to continue riding social cooperation to higher levels of stability and complexity. But to what end? Perhaps to expand the reach of wisdom and virtue wherever and whenever the possibility to do so had evolved.

John F. Haught is the Distinguished Research Professor in the Department of Theology at Georgetown University. In his essay "Purpose in Nature," he develops a more open-minded synthesis of ideas pertaining to the false dichotomy of God versus evolution:

> I believe we must expand our vision from one that focuses narrowly on biological evolution and ask about the wider *universe* that sponsors the Darwinian process. Life and evolution, after all, are features of a much larger cosmos than the rather restricted territory that evolutionary naturalists typically take into account...Naturalists, as I read them, usually conflate the notion of purpose with that of "intelligent design"...however, from a religious or theological view, purpose is not the same thing as design...I take purpose to mean not design but an *overall aim toward the actualizing of value*...To understand

the *real* world, I suggest, we need to attend carefully not only to the objectifiable world but also to the reality of our own inner experience. After all, our own experience and conscious-ness are not alien to nature...each one of us, including the sci-entist, already knows that subjective experience—our own as well as that of many other living beings—is a fact of nature.

Haught quotes the geologist, paleontologist, and religious thinker Pierre Teilhard de Chardin, from his book *The Human Phenomenon*:

The time has come for us to realize that to be satisfactory, any interpretation of the universe...must cover the inside as well as the outside of things—spirit as well as matter. True physics is that which will someday succeed in integrating the totality of the human being into a coherent representation of the world.

Haught puts forward that "Cosmic purpose may be coexten-sive with, though not reducible to, the long story of nature's grad-ually intensifying its insideness or subjectivity." In its search for meaning, evolving intelligence moves from a lopsided regard for objective analyses toward more incorporation of subjective syn-theses. This trend is prompted by the perceived need to process what's going on in the fully integrated whole of our experience in reality. It also hints that the higher forms of wisdom and vir-tue needed to sponsor health and sustainability require subjective input.

On Earth the cosmic story witnessed the emergence of the human subplot, which has *Homo sapiens* racing to solve the puzzle of its existence while finding a sustainable way of living before it's too late. At the same time new principles of human health and wellness are coming to light. This includes the principle of working narrative into the healing process. In a narrative with a long arc there are many chapters. Some of these chapters are bleak and filled with evil, death, and suffering. But in the end, it is not what a given chapter is about that matters; what matters is what the story will be about. Writes Haught:

> What requires understanding is the delicate blend of openness, constraint, and temporality that clothes the cosmos in the apparel of drama...We shall never get to the bottom of evolution until we have understood why nature is open to narrative in the first place.

Clinical problem solving begins with assessment. Patient care starts with a careful construction of the patient's health narrative. In the care of all living systems, clinical assessment also depends on narrative for context and for clues concerning what health and sustainability requires. This is why Dr. V placed so much emphasis on trying to construct a narrative for life on Earth that all people could relate to.

From detailed narratives emerge hints as to the gist of what's going right or wrong, and what can be done to turn a story of health decaying to illness into a story of wellness restored and maintained. Only from increasingly refined working explanations of what's going on will we find the deep clinical solutions to our root problems.

Narrative-based integrative medicine is an ongoing, zoom in/pan back, left-brain/right-brain process of analysis and pattern recognition, aimed at getting the facts straight so we can understand what the story means and make good judgments about what to do. For complex clinical dilemmas, this is our way of trying to fully understand the problem before jumping to its solution.

Consulting a patient is, for both the clinical systems biologist and the planetary medicine specialist—nothing more than a quest to translate findings into functional integration and positive meaning—accomplish that much, and health and sustainability may just take care of themselves.

Imagine humanity getting two specialist opinions on its health from planetary medicine doctors who practice elsewhere in the Milky Way. Humanity's goal in getting these opinions is to build functional integrity and expand access to positive meaning. The evidence-based approach of the gene-centered naturalist might go something like this:

Hello, humanity? This is Dr. Stoneman from Galactic Certainty. The reports on the Earth system are back. Looks like you serve no purpose other than being a vehicle for genes competing to avoid the title of "weakest link." You're on your last chance. It's investigational and there are real risks but you might prolong your survival with a species-wide transplant of stem cells modified to contain genes designed to promote altruism and social cooperation. In fact we just had another species cancel. We could do yours next week. Can you scrape up the funds? If not we can loan you the money at a reasonable rate when you take into account that your survival is at stake. What do you think?

The narrative-based approach of the clinical systems biologist might go something like this:

Hello, humanity? This is Dr. Bickerson from Planetary Medical. I've looked at your lab results, and, to be honest, you're in a bit of a pickle. You really ought to put some effort into getting faith and reason on the same page. You'll get more mileage from your genes *and* your social efforts to fit into the bigger scheme of things on that beautiful planet of yours. You should meet with our lifestyle change coordinator.

With that impressive prefrontal cortex of yours, I'm sure y'all can find a way to regulate those darn fears and urges and make it work.

Narrative-based assessment insists on not cutting itself off from the deep complexity of what's going on within the living system that is you. Why should we be any less careful not to cut ourselves off from the deep complexity of what's going on within the living system that is *us*?

Scientific reasoning is justifiably wary of oversimplification—until it reaches the limits of objectivity, at which point it likes to cut itself loose from subjectivity as if it were a lethal poison. On the sufficiency of evolutionary naturalism as a worldview, Haught concludes:

> The naturalistic enshrinement of either chance or necessity can survive only in an illusory and imaginative world of ideas quite cut off from the actual narrative flow of nature and of life itself. And this narrative, a story that wends we know not where, may for all we know be pregnant with the promise of ultimate meaning. If so, there may still be abundant room, alongside of science, for a theology of evolution.

This is perhaps the take-home point for *Homo sapiens*, a species that, despite being in distress remains overly infatuated with itself. As Professor Haught cautions, perhaps the essential ingredients of evolution—substance, energy, information, chance, selection, and cosmic stretches of time—are interacting to propel the unfolding narrative of the cosmos in a direction pregnant with meaning.

Indeed, thus far, it can be argued, the evolutionary narrative contains a leitmotif of major transitions. But the ingredients of the cosmos did not create evolution; they simply appeared, in a process that remains shrouded in mystery—quantum physical hypotheses for how something came from nothing notwithstanding. Wisdom is a product of evolution, but evolution is a product of creation. The source of all wisdom is the creation mystery.

The narrative of evolutionary biology moves against chaos toward systems that are more complex and functional. The narrative now seems to depend less on genes than on the ability of subjectively derived meaning to foster enhanced social cooperation. If you will, a subjectively derived but objectively measurable sense of purpose and direction is emerging as a new dynamic in social evolution. We endanger our ability to fulfill this purpose without integration between faith and reason and a more balanced relationship between heart and mind.

Creation is the source of all wisdom, and the how and why of creation has yet to be limited to our scientific understanding of it. This is why Dr. V's team felt that theological reasoning deserves a seat at any table where the agenda under discussion concerns health and sustainability.

Gaining a seat at the health and sustainability table is not an invitation for theologians to expect nonbelievers to accept their metaphysical assumptions. Rather, it is an invitation for theology to contribute to the clinical task of moving cultures toward the social cooperation required to create health and sustainability.

Absolutism has no place in attempts to fashion clinical solutions to complex problems. Absolutist visions are necessarily subjective, as there are no objective grounds for absolute truth; absolutist visions have a perfect track record for underestimating the complexity of reality. We must be on guard to avoid overreaching when making claims about human nature, the truth, reality, or the way things ought to be.

From a clinical perspective, in light of where evolution seems to want to go, a split between faith and reason cannot be considered wise. Nor can faith or reason without humility be considered wise. Premature certainty about fundamental beliefs suppresses social cooperativeness.

If our clinical philosophy guides us to seek genuine wisdom (and it does), then we must undertake the quest with humility and candor. Cultural diversity is what it is, making cultural change is a tall order, but there is no path to health and sustainability that does not involve cultural change.

Under these conditions, an integrative clinical mind-set calls for a fresh commitment to intellectual integrity. We will not locate genuine wisdom if we lose sight of the fact that creation, the source of all wisdom, remains shrouded in mystery.

We are less likely to achieve health and sustainability in a world whose cultures separate faith from reason, or pit one faith against another. We cannot find wellness by splitting objective from subjective experience as if one were the king of all knowledge and the other a motley fool. Since there is no objective proof for or against the existence of God, we are left with the *possibility* of God—and all the richness of meaning that this implies.

In *Ethics from a Theocentric Perspective*, James Gustafson cautioned readers to let God be God—that God will not be manipulated, ignored, or denied. Viewing ethics from a health and sustainability perspective, it seems practical to apply the same reasoning to a weaker proposition by saying, *Let the possibility of God be the possibility of God, and do not let this possibility be manipulated, ignored, or denied.* The God idea is not dead—it is pregnant with the meaning that, for all we know, the universe has a Maker.

From a clinical standpoint, an intelligent species that responds in a fitting way to the possibility of God is one giant step closer to finding its way to health and sustainability—assuming it can cleave to good faith and good religion.

The implications for the clinical philosophy of health and sustainability under construction here are intriguing. They involve a simultaneous commitment to two ways of understanding the world:

1. A radically empirical understanding of both the objective and subjective facets of human existence, known as *radical empiricism*.

2. A program for understanding evolution that finds room for the possibility of God, known as *theistic evolution*.

Radical empiricism asserts that any serious worldview must take into account both the objective world of physical reality and the subjective world of meaning. Theistic evolution postulates God to be the force behind the creation of the natural universe, wherein nature creates complexity through laws of evolution that come to point in the direction of wisdom, virtue, and increasingly fitting ways of responding to a Maker.

Together, these two philosophical commitments lay the foundation for a worldview that Dr. V refers to as *idealistic realism*—the clinically most robust worldview from which to approach a move toward health and sustainability because the roots of health and sustainability can thrive in the ground of radical empiricism and theistic evolution.

Agreements on policy details are made more likely as neither faith nor reason has hegemony over the direction of cultural growth and change. A higher form of functional integration emerges, marking a path toward social cooperation.

The laws of evolution venture beyond chance, necessity, and the depth of evolutionary time by allowing for the emergence of unpredictable new mechanisms as systems add complexity. Earth's dominant animal has an opportunity to will a more functional level of social cooperation into being. Dr. V and her team wanted to help the species seize this opportunity.

The predictable laws of evolution and the unpredictable turns of emergence converge on fundamental functional solutions to problems of species adaptation that repeatedly entail social group formation, maintenance, and transformation—processes that require increasingly complex and functional forms of social cooperation.

As a species we seem to be converging toward an idealistic realism that can climb its way to health and sustainability, because along this path, new solutions to cultural change will emerge in ways that are natural and consistent with past examples of major transitions in social evolution. Imagine what the next round of social cooperation and transformation could do with a globally distributed network of social media. The game's not over, folks.

But creationists be forewarned: theistic evolution is not to be confused with creationism in any way, shape, or form. Theistic evolution accepts the findings of methodologically sound science. It is silent when asked to show objective evidence for God's ability or desire to intervene in a way that supersedes the laws of nature. The primary function of theistic evolution is to remind us that when it comes to a Maker, or the existence of one true God, absence of evidence is not evidence of absence.

Our cultures find convincing objective support for evolution, and strong subjective support for viewing evolution as an unfolding narrative that, at the very least, cannot dismiss a theological context for creation. This cast of idealistic realism views faith and reason as strategic partners in an effort to discern a path to sustainability. It is not derived through analytical philosophy. Rather, it naturally emerges as an extension of a narrative-hungry clinical philosophy whose purpose is to heal and sustain.

The intention of the healer is to explain something not for its own sake, but in order to heal something. The motives are ideal-driven, but the search for explanatory power is driven by logic and scientific method as far as the healer can take them; after that, it is experience and intuition all the way down.

Philosopher Nicholas Rescher addresses the topic of idealistic realism in *The Blackwell Guide to Metaphysics*. He notes that for thinking creatures, the "real world" has two key dimensions: physical and mental. We generally accept that physical reality exists independently of the minds that study it. We also accept that our mental interpretations of reality are part of reality as well, and that our interpretations of the real world can influence how the physical and mental dimensions of the real world evolve.

Rescher points out that communication simply doesn't work unless we have a way to agree about the available facts of physical reality. For example, the facts of biological reality are the ultimate arbiters of the adequacy of our theorizing about medical care or the sustainability of our species.

While the difference between reality itself and our mental picture of it is vast, we nonetheless benefit from our scientific understanding of the physical world.

Mental reality, on the other hand, is subjective and hard to render into factual statements. Reaching conceptual agreement is more difficult than coming to agreement about physical facts, yet mental reality is no less part of the whole than its physical counterpart. Unless we have a way to fundamentally agree about our mental experience, we may cease communicating and lose our opportunities for finding a cooperative path to health and sustainability.

Rescher argues that we accept what physical reality is like in order to learn more about what we *should do with it*. That is to say, the rationale for accepting scientific theory lies within a larger framework of purpose supplied by the mind. In this view, our commitment to a reality that exists independently from the mind arises not *from* experience but *for* it. He concludes, "Realism is a position to which we are constrained not by the push of evidence but by the pull of purpose."

Our ideals are conceived on the subjective side of reality, where the facts don't add up but the meaning makes sense—sometimes enough sense to be affirmed as wisdom. The tools of science help us make sense of the objective side of reality, where the facts add up but the meaning's not clear. It is easier to reach agreement when we've justified a decision based on clear scientific evidence. But agreeing about which ideals to place highest is notoriously difficult, even when health and sustainability are at stake. Yet the ideals of health, wellness, and the sustainability of life strongly resonate with people of all cultures, especially when the going gets tough.

The idealistic realism Dr. V proposed can be viewed as a branch of clinical philosophy whose "pull of purpose" comes from a desire for health and sustainability, and whose "push of evidence" orients us to help solve the puzzle of how to get there.

If a physician commits to helping a patient as a whole person, there is no choice but to integrate the objective realm of biology with the subjective realm of the mind and its psychosocial dynamics. There is no choice but to become a clinical systems biologist who can move between these realms, zooming in to the molecular level here, panning back to the psychosocial level there.

Were the patient a developing world system, a planetary medicine doctor would approach it with the same philosophy applied to a wider narrative: attain wisdom in systems biology *and* cultural dynamics, and apply this wisdom with a purpose to heal.

The theological position built into this form of idealistic realism is clinically necessary. From the standpoint of planetary medicine, good theology lends the human search for meaning a powerful sense of purpose and a much-needed dose of humility.

Theology has been upstaged by science; it deserves a more prominent role in the human drama. The swell of scientific support for the idea that evolution converges on certain categories of functional adaptation indicates that evolution is at least partly purpose-driven. This is theology's cue to rejoin science at center stage.

The idea of evolutionary convergence stems from the observation that species whose genetic lineages branched away from each other in the distant past nonetheless evolve the same basic solutions to puzzles dealing with matters of function and adaptation. Since this concept of convergent evolution has proponents and critics, it should be considered unproven, though it is under serious investigation.

Evolution appears to converge when different genes from different species follow different pathways to arrive at the same functional solution. In this case, genes become the means by which nature moves complex systems toward narrow sets of solutions to problems of adaptation. Put differently, some genetic solutions appear to evolve in parallel as opposed to one long branching

series. Yet the parallel solutions still seem to conform to prede-
termined specifications. In this sense, genetic evolution seems to
converge in a particular direction.

University of Cambridge paleontologist Simon Conway
Morris is a thought leader on the subject of evolutionary convergence. In *The Deep Structure of Biology*, he moves from the biological evidence to the wider implications of a convergent evolution.

For example, molecules called opsins have become part of
the solution by which insect and animal species solve the problem of being able to see things. They reached these solutions
through what appear to be distinct evolutionary branch points
and pathways.

But molecular solutions are not the only things converging
as evolution marches through time; intelligence is also on the
move. Conway Morris explains, "If evolution has a spectrum of
discussion, and one end point is molecular, the other is the level
of complexity that is a prerequisite of intelligences that will lead
to self-knowledge and ethical action." He explores three biological properties at the complex end of the spectrum: mammal-ness,
brains, and mentalities.

Before mammals appeared, there was a species that bridged
monitor-like reptiles and mammals. Functionally adaptive traits
held by a range of different species emerged along this bridge;
these include courtship behavior, hunting, and intelligent social
structures.

Also noteworthy are the physiological, mental, and social
similarities between birds and mammals. Similarities include
warm-bloodedness, parental caring instincts, group social behaviors that include cooperative hunting and social play, and sophisti-

cated vocalizations, music-making, tool-making, and the cultural transmission of vocal signaling and problem-solving concepts.

The differences among land-, air-, and water-based intelligences are revealed somewhat in their brain structures. Primates, wolves, crows, dolphins, and whales have each worked out their own unique anatomical and chemical brain property sets, but in notable ways their evolving mentalities converge around particular solutions to functional adaptation puzzles. Conway Morris writes:

> If evolution is effectively the motor whereby the deeper realities of the universe may be uncovered, then it might be that an idealistic program can help to expel the corrosive relativism that attempts to etch our framework of meaning.

> Science necessarily works in a naturalistic framework, but the identification of any principle immediately begs foundational issues...It is worth recalling that the suspicion of a metaphysic in biology, with the consequent abandonment of any search for deeper meanings, has an alarming counterpart in the humanities. In a framework where language (and music) is regarded as a mere evolutionary accident, is it so surprising that the humanities can be so readily poisoned and corrupted by the postmodernist enterprise?

By fragmenting human experience into isolated cells, where reason occupies one floor, faith another, with the humanities relegated to a corner of the basement, we're placing bars and walls between the objective and subjective parts of the universe. We lose flexibility for solving the problems of humanity when our thought processes are housed in a prison of our own making.

The implications of convergent evolution go deeper than the reconciliation of science with philosophy, theology, ethics, and the arts. Conway Morris writes:

> If the mind is adaptive to a real universe constrained by natural law, then the search for extraterrestrial intelligence is not an absurd gamble but as strong a prediction as finding that the long sought-after sentient extraterrestrial is looking at us with camera eyes.

The kind of camera eyes that evolved in thousands of ways in species on Earth, different in terms of molecular detail but identical in terms of the function served—the ability to see what needs to be seen in order to survive—are the kinds of camera eyes we can expect to find in any other galaxy.

All of the eyes, capable of evolving anywhere in this universe, will be more similar than different to Carl Sagan's eyes as he looked into the camera to ask, "Who speaks for Earth?"

They will be more similar than different to Jacob Bronowski's eyes as he looked away from the camera to a handful of mud from the grounds at Auschwitz, lamenting the sterility of science by the numbers, hoping for a way to place science back in relationship to the humanities, where it can relearn how to touch people.

Carl Sagan (1934-1996) and Jacob Bronowski (1908-1974) spoke eloquently about the fact that reality is always more complex than we think it is. If you want to be in charge, start your own universe. We don't make the rules; we discern them. Only through a blend of our best science, our most stirring works of art, and our wisest and most inspirational visionaries can we learn what functional adaptations creation—and perhaps a Creator—press upon us. As much as we need them, good ideas are not enough. We also need engineers of cultural change to help them work.

This is how a planetary medicine doctor came to wonder whether a collectively felt sense of ethical responsibility, acted upon and aimed at promoting health and wellness within living systems and in human affairs, is the modern adaptation upon which creation would have our species converge at this moment in history on Earth.

This convergent solution would apply to all planet-plundering species of life in the universe as they try to work their way out of the pickles they're in. In addition to camera-like eyes, evolution might also reward intelligent species that learn to leave their cultural intolerances at the door so they can cooperate in solving their health and sustainability problems. Adaptation on the part of our species cannot occur without a willingness to entertain a new mix of analyses and syntheses built on the shoulders of our best wisdom and virtues so far.

Aiming to realize an ideal is like setting a treatment goal— the results are better if you've first obtained a detailed narrative and some good working explanations for what's going on. The science of complexity may have more questions than answers at this point, but it's on the right paradigm-changing track.

Complex systems science underscores the limits of reductionism. It is changing the way we think about the driving mechanisms of evolution, and it is foraging through multiple disciplines to discover the mathematics of organized complexity, which promises to be different than any current mathematical way of describing what nature is up to.

The science of complexity points us in a new direction that feels right to a growing number of scientists and theologians from a growing number of disciplines, but the picture remains blurry. So with humility we set off into the last remaining deep wilderness on planet Earth—human nature—where we will gather more clues about what, besides gene selection, evolution may be up to.

A Creation in
Search of Stewards

◇◇◇◇◇◇◇◇◇◇◇◇◇◇◇◇◇◇◇◇◇◇◇◇◇◇◇◇◇◇◇◇◇◇◇◇

All narratives have the mystery of creation as prologue. This mystery pulses through every element of every story ever told. As Carl Sagan put it, "If you want to make an apple pie truly from scratch, first you must invent the universe."

Many students are challenged to reconcile their inherited religious worldviews with the teachings of science. When people growing up in homes with literalist religious beliefs encounter the facts of natural history, the resulting cognitive dissonance can lead them to one of three ways of coping:

1. Form split worldviews, one based on scientific knowledge, the other on religious beliefs. This is the twenty-first-century schizoid option.

2. Choose between worldviews by abandoning science or abandoning religion. This is the frontal lobe ablation option.

3. Integrate the two worldviews into a coherent whole, in which science and religious belief are no longer viewed as contradictory. This is the health and sustainability plan.

Pew surveys of religious belief among the American public and members of the American Academy of Science, showed the following results:

	The Public	Scientists
Believe in God	83%	33%
Don't believe in God, but believe in a universal spirit or higher power	12%	18%
Don't believe in either	4%	41%
Don't know or refused to answer	1%	7%

Source: Scientists data from Pew Research Center for the People & Press survey conducted in May and June 2009. General public data from Pew Research Center survey conducted in July 2006.

Almost half of the public and scientists polled don't believe in God or a higher power—which isn't to say they can't live meaningful and happy lives. Over half of the scientists polled believe in God or a higher power, showing their ability to integrate the sacred with the secular. If 83 percent of the public believes in God but only 33 percent of scientists do, scientific training appears to lead a chunk of the public to drop their belief in God. What's unclear is how many scientists move from atheism to belief in God.

We know it happens. Ask Francis Collins, the physician-geneticist who led the Human Genome Project to triumph and, as of this writing, directs the National Institutes of Health. Widely respected in the community of scientific elites, Collins converted to Christianity after many years of atheism. In his book *The Language of God*, Collins takes the position that "science is not threatened by God; it is enhanced." In his book *Belief: Readings on the Reason for Faith*, he explores philosophical, theological, social, and ethical points of view from esteemed thinkers who were able to integrate faith and reason into a single worldview without imploding.

If you look into the much-publicized culture war between science and religion, you see that it is driven in large part by small bands of dogmatists bending and shaping facts and opinions to fit what they want to believe.

Theistic evolutionists steer clear of the crossfire and go about their business accepting that science and evolution are real but are only part of a story that makes room for the possibility that we have a Maker to whom we are accountable. Billions of human beings experience gut-level certainty that God exists. That fact doesn't make it so, but it is a fact that's relevant to any attempt by global institutions and leaders to find a path toward health and sustainability.

For science, religion, and every other human way of construing the meaning of the world and our role in it, reality, thus far, keeps proving to be more complex than we thought.

In *Complexity*, Melanie Mitchell calls attention to a fundamental problem we have in predicting the behavior of complex systems, known as *sensitive dependence on initial conditions*, or the *butterfly effect*. In any complex system of multiple interacting

components, even the tiniest variation in the initial conditions
can produce massive differences in the subsequent behavior of the
system, making that behavior hard to predict.

Humanity's industrial presence on the planet constitutes a
particular set of initial conditions that will determine the degree
of freedom that future generations will have to find solutions to
their problems. Each set of living generations sits at the controls of cultural and technological evolution. What we do with
these controls will determine whether future generations look
back on us with gratitude or disdain. From where we sit, our
progress toward health and sustainability is hard to predict.
Whether it is a patient or a planet with complex health problems that are not fully understood, the clinically wise course is
to assume neither the worst nor the best while continuing to dig
for solutions aimed at restoring functional integrity to the system
as a whole.

When it comes to assessing and treating chronic illness, it
is prudent to avoid snap judgments and to maintain an open
mind; complexity demands this of the healer. Complexity would
demand the same cautious and open-minded humility from those
who would lead cultural change interventions aimed at long-term
wellness.

How then, do science and religion measure up as humble
guides to wisdom and virtue along the cultural change route to
health and sustainability? Each of these great pillars of culture
could be doing a much better job of helping humans cope with
reality on reality's terms.

Look more closely at a pillar of culture and you will actually
see a dynamic web of subcultures in a constant state of interaction.
At any given time, various subcultures are working to change

the world but making little headway except for those pulling the strings that control campaign financing. As an example, let's look at what America's Christian subcultures have accomplished in their efforts to change American culture.

It is fair to say that American culture is pluralistic without a coherent worldview that truly captures the diverse sentiments of the hearts and minds that make up the nation as a whole. The American public approached this sense of unity in diversity after 9/11, but it quickly decayed into partisan political rancor. The opportunity passed, and so did the public's chance of changing the political dynamics of America's political institutions.

The efforts of subcultures to take control of American culture are ongoing. One of the most visible signs is the culture war that pits a secular, progressive America against a religious, conservative America, each with its own set of allies in the media.

The atmosphere created by these media is rich with innuendo, drive-by character assassination, and finger pointing. In these settings, values and ethics are mere props in bad plays about new visions for America. Meanwhile, church membership is declining across America. This is in part because American society is growing more pluralistic. So many new subcultures are sprouting up in an already-crowded field that it is no longer realistic to think that any of these subcultures can ascend to a position where it can persuade a majority of Americans to adopt its worldview.

Even if an American subculture emerged with a worldview and the institutional power to change what Americans believe and how they behave, newer worldviews would keep popping up in the market of alternatives. The current king of worldviews in the game of thrones would face nonstop competition, in addition to nonstop harassment, from other groups vying for the crown.

James Davison Hunter's work *To Change the World* is subtitled *The Irony, Tragedy, and Possibility of Christianity in the Late Modern World*. Hunter is a good social scientist and a Christian who understands why the conservative and liberal wings of Christian culture are failing to change the overall course of American society.

"Christians," writes Hunter, "as a rule, are nothing if not sincere." Their hearts are in the right place, but their minds have too shallow a grasp on the dynamics of change in a society that is growing more fragmented and diverse by the minute.

Christians on the right and left side of the spectrum conceive and pursue their cultural change efforts using distinctive political theologies. Conservative Christian political theology engages American culture with an approach that too angrily defends against what it perceives to be the major sins of secular culture. The right to choose an abortion, use embryonic stem cells, even to be gay or lesbian, let alone engage in same-sex marriage—these are viewed as assaults on biblical tradition and the institution of the family. In the process, conservative Christians appear to undervalue the biblical traditions of social service and justice, and the global imperative to become better stewards of the planet, instead resorting to bullying tactics that would break the heart of Jesus.

Progressive Christian political theology engages American culture with an approach that too readily amends tradition in an attempt to remain more relevant to secular culture. For the sake of secular culture, they're more willing to question orthodoxy and to downplay conservative social values in return for greater commitments to social justice, service to others, and environmental activism. In the process, progressive Christians appear as traitors to the long-standing efforts of conservative

Christians to defend America against the breakdown of its traditional values.

Both wings of Christian political theology in America fall prey to their own idealism. The conservatives have mastered the art of naming enemies and politicizing their cause. They appear strong, and this helps them believe that they are somehow winning the culture war that they started. The progressives have mastered the art of meekness. They're more willing to consort with secularists because both groups know what it's like to be demonized by the more rabid voices of the Christian right.

Needless to say, polarized American Christianity is having a hard time breaking out of its own subcultures with any kind of compelling vision for leading America through the tough times that realists see on the horizon, rapidly heading our way.

The world scientific community, however, is busy organizing a rational response to a growing set of social, political, economic, and environmental threats to health and sustainability. These threats include widespread poverty, hunger, and infectious disease, climate change, ocean acidification, pollution, loss of biodiversity, energy and water shortages, natural disasters, and so on. Religious missions also initiate relief efforts, lending considerable hands to the relief of human suffering. Millionaire preachers and the largesse of the Church distract from the efforts of small but courageous faith-based outfits operating on shoestring budgets, just as the science-industrial complex casts its shadow over the courageous healing intent of the secular not-for-profits that tend to the sick, hungry, and poor.

The international scientific community seems, on the whole, more interested than the international religious community in the safety and welfare of the Earth system. Educated people around the world have growing concerns about our ability to manage the many threats to our health and sustainability. They yearn to see physicians, scientists, and religious folk join together to create a culture of urgency about these problems, including our biggest health and sustainability dilemma: elevating the standard of living for the poor without plundering or poisoning the planet.

Yet within archconservative American political theology, scientists are viewed as part of the secularization problem that needs to be defended against, as if evolution and climate change are nothing more than the syphilitic secular dreams of godless scientists. The irony lies in thinking that a political theology of American exceptionalism can win a sustainable influence on the nation's culture by passing out blinders against science. This antirealism masquerading as idealism would lead our species in a direction opposite to health and sustainability and, presumably, away from what God would desire for humankind.

Hunter details the perils of idealism when applied to the business of changing cultures:

> Idealism ignores the way culture is generated, coordinated, and organized. Thus, it underrates how difficult it is to penetrate culture and influence its direction. Idealism leads to a naïveté about the nature of culture and its dynamics that is, in the end, fatal.

> Culture is much less an invention of the will than it is a slow product of history. It organizes a way of being, and not just a course of action, and it does so in a way that makes our understanding of the world seem natural. It takes shape in a concrete institutional form...and exists at the interface between ideas and institutions.

Hunter disputes the "great-man view of history and culture," in which societies are led forth by heroic individuals of prodigious vision and talent:

> The key actor in history is not individual genius but rather the network and the new institutions that are created out of those networks. And the more "dense" the network—that is, the more active and interactive the network—the more influential it could be. This is where the stuff of culture and cultural change is produced.

In describing the anatomical features of culture, Hunter shows why people within any given culture are unable to achieve a unified, fully coherent worldview:

> Culture also is composed of innumerable *fields*—relatively distinct and often-overlapping regions of meaning, activity, networks, and relationships, as well as rules and interests. Religious traditions and ideological movements can be thought of as fields of culture as can publishing, entertainment, education, ministry, and the like. Each of these has it's own range of subfields. By their very nature, these too have their own logic, dynamics, and direction, as well as their own center and periphery.

> Beyond all of this there are the relatively distinct, often competing perspectives that are drawn from different geological regions of a society, various ethnic groups and social classes, and an infinite range of religious traditions and moral communities. For these reasons, culture, especially in the modern world, can never be fully coherent.

Hunter does not intend to underplay the role of individuals, as they are often the ones supplying the vision, the funding, and the credibility needed to get new networks off the ground; individuals form the "connective tissue of the network itself."

Andy Crouch is a Christian writer who comes at cultural change from a different angle. In his book *Culture Making: Recovering Our Creative Calling*, he writes:

> Culture changes when people actually make more and better culture. If we want to transform culture, what we actually have to do is get into the midst of the human cultural product and create some new cultural goods that reshape the way people imagine and experience their world.

In other words, those who want to change culture need to dive into it and emerge with some new creations that build traction for their cause. Dive into culture, and you'll find a rich mix of science, religion, markets, professions, governments, news and the media, technology, engineering, fashion, design, food and agriculture, sport and recreation, language, literature, poetry, music, film, dance, theatre, painting, sculpture, photography, and so on.

Crouch reasons that there is a strategy to Christian culture making: create new cultural goods that can capture imaginations and win hearts and minds to the example of Jesus.

Hunter counters that when it comes to changing culture, heart-and-mind strategies often prove futile:

> They fail to recognize and address the relationship of culture to the dynamics and structures of power that operate in the world (and in the culture itself).

In other words, it takes more than sincerity or market popularity for new cultural goods to change the larger culture in any deep historical sense. The larger culture is so complex that it won't take directions. You cannot lead it by the nose because it doesn't

have a face—it has millions of faces. This point persuaded Dr. V
and her team that the best they could hope to do was keep nudg-
ing it until its forms and functions reorganize to a point where
the ideals of health and sustainability are within realistic reach.

Hunter is all in favor of new cultural ideas and products that
can inspire hearts and minds, but he wants a sober clinical assessment of the challenge that awaits culture makers:

> While we all share the imperative to be culture makers, we
> finally cannot change the world because we cannot anticipate
> or dictate how any cultural artifact will be accepted by others.

Cultural change artists must extend their reach not just into
various subcultures, fields, and subfields but also into the institutions that influence what's going on in these cultural compart-
ments. The connective tissue of culture includes institutions and
the elite groups that lead them and that wield considerable political and financial power. Though we should not discount what
empowered individuals can accomplish, empowered networks
have a better chance of influencing change agents. What's needed
in order to change culture is something like a clinical strategy
based on idealistic realism that can mobilize social networks to
achieve cultural change at institutional levels. The modern quest
for health and sustainability is not a spectator sport—it is an
audience participation exercise that continues until the forces of
health and sustainability win or lose.

In modern America, any participants in the various fields and
subfields of Christian culture, attempting to change the values and
activities of American culture, would be wise to study Hunter's
work, which amounts to a general and systematic overview of the
physiology of culture.

Crouch's advice to make culture by producing cultural goods that inspire people to lives of virtue also has an important role to play. If necessity is the mother of invention, perhaps inspiration is the father of intention.

Christians in America would also do well to heed John Armstrong's call for the Catholic, Protestant, and Eastern Orthodox institutional giants of Christian culture to join in principle, and to network their institutions around their sacred shared belief that, first and foremost, the human path should be lit and inspired by the teachings of Jesus. Without such collaboration, the Christian tradition could amount to window dressing in a world whose science education and research enterprise keep gaining adherents by force of logic.

In a fully integrated network of cultural systems, the humble scientist will not cringe at the idea of subjectively anchored forms of logic, and the humble believer will not cringe at the idea of faith grounded in the facts of evolution and environmental change.

Collective wisdom should be grounded in the idea that we're not *entirely sure* why the universe happened, although we're *reasonably sure* of how it has been operating since moments after the Big Bang. Religious traditions that want to remain relevant ignore the facts of evolution at their own risk; they must be free to ask, "Given that, now what?"

Wisdom traditions cannot live on science alone. They combine logic, scientific method, values, and subjective experience in their attempts to link statements about what *is* with statements about what *ought to be*. As Jacob Bronowski lamented, science and logic are unable to link meaning with moral value in a coherent way without the help of wisdom that dares to associate with things metaphysical. Science and logic cannot be the sole arbiters of human wisdom. They lack the emotional power of the humanities and their artistic and spiritual inspirations. From a clinical standpoint, inspiration is as necessary as food and water to human flourishing.

When an integrative clinical mind-set asks the clinical question, "What's going on?" it does so with a mission to find answers that will promote health and wellness. The mission of the physician is not to find a diagnosis and slap a treatment into place—it is to explain how a given illness narrative points to what a particular sufferer needs to regain functional integrity and remain a capable and inspired person in the world.

This clinical problem-solving method is patterned closely on scientific method—but with the important exception that, where complex chronic illness is involved, it must consult the subjective world of human experience, where history taking and narrative construction require additional time on the part of the physician. Yet if a clinical problem solver uses experience and intuition to diverge from usual and customary care, the health insurer can deem the service "medically unnecessary" or "investigational" and therefore not covered under the patient's health benefits structure. It is a sign of sickness within the medical culture that physicians must summon the courage to heal using subjective experience in spite of a health plan's unwillingness to pay for this form of expertise.

These insurance tactics are justified when a physician's divergent use of experience and intuition benefits no one but himself. But insurers also use these tactics to bully physicians into adopting a herd mentality that leaves many patients with chronic illness alone in the room because the doctor ran out of time. Physicians who stray from the herd to help these patients can become prey, even if their divergent path leads to the kind of functional innovation that our health system screams for.

The false dichotomies between the objective and the subjective are not the only ones we need to heal. The sham split between faith and reason, and between medical intuition and medical logic, are examples of a forced separation between *description* and *prescription*. On our quest for health and sustainability, the famous dialectic between *is* and *ought* will warrant our reconsideration.

Philosophers have struggled for centuries to find graceful ways by which to move from statements about *what is* to statements about *what ought to be*. Since the Enlightenment period, most have had their analytical heads removed with a guillotine built by the British Moralist David Hume, as presented in his book *An Inquiry Concerning the Principles of Morals*.

Hume argued that the logic of the moral senses and the logic of the rational mind are two different species of being, and that any attempt to mate them will fail because reality has already chopped them into irreconcilable categories of experience.

Maybe—maybe not. As time passes and new things are learned, new complexities and ambiguities creep into the mix. If we insert into the "no ought from is" debate the bodymind wisdom rule that reality is always more complex than we think it is, there is a consequence for clinical problem solvers. In the face of nature's ineffable complexity, we need an integrative clinical mind-set that counsels us to tolerate ambiguity and imprecision, to take full advantage of our experience and intuitive logic rather than jump to conclusions that are hard and fast but potentially wrong and unsafe.

Rules-based algorithms have their place in acute, emergency, intensive, and surgical forms of care, but they are not enough when it comes to solving the puzzles posed by chronic illness, where the problems are extraordinarily complex. Better here to invest in a clinical mind-set that asks us to put up with the frailty of human logic accepting that nature follows *its* logic, not ours— and thus far, nature's logic continually proves to be more complex than we thought it was. Chronic illnesses reflect this complexity, whether they occur in organisms, in markets, or in cultures.

We should be humble about our attempts to *prove* where a line might be drawn between logic, math, physics, and reason on one side, and a feelings-driven human sense of judgment and morality on the other. When using an integrative clinical mind-set to assess chronically ill systems, established proofs and evidence-based guidelines never carry enough authority to close doors to further clinical inquiry.

At best, high quality scientific evidence offers but a tentative answer to a still-ambiguous question. Where the wellness of a living system is at stake, fully solved equations matter less than finding a path to whatever works. When a wellness goal is achieved, it is easy to live with the critics who protest that we have yet to connect enough dots to explain how the method worked.

It serves little purpose to get bogged down in the technicalities of arguments so resistant to settlement when all around us we find urgent needs to adapt to the requirements of health and wellness.

Echoing the Greek philosophers, the Spanish-American philosopher George Santayana (1863–1952) wrote, "reality means what the intellect infers from the data of sense." In other words, reality is what it is, but it means whatever our senses and reasoning capacity together decide it should mean.

In *The Life of Reason*, Santayana writes of how human senses and an ability to manipulate symbols gave birth to the faculty of reason. A philosopher by trade, he expressed ideas more like an artist flirting with a muse. His theme in this work was to trace the life of reason from its birth into its modern, childlike state.

Santayana felt that the life of reason illustrated and foreshadowed the "unity given to all existence by a mind *in love with the good.*" This notion offers a means by which to understand how *is* becomes *ought* on the time scale of evolution. Santayana claims that from its very beginning, reason was not a function of logic, but of wisdom that combines logic with values.

Reality doesn't slow down to see whether human logic has proven how to move from *is* to *ought*; it just keeps flowing. When reason finally comes of age in our heads, it will understand that the rational mind falls short of wisdom if it bars intuition, imagination, art, passion, and faith from entry into the conversation. Reason will have finally matured when it can combine the emotional input of human experience with its logically grounded interpretations. Only then will it be capable of wisdom that supports health and sustainability. The "science reveals that life has no inherent purpose" crowd will then see their own grotesque reflections in Quixote's battered helmet.

Santayana was an atheist who insisted that religions "are the great fairy-tales of the conscience." He joined Kant in despising dogmatic religious traditions that anoint themselves as guardians of literal and absolute truth while proceeding on paths of self-aggrandizement.

However, like Kant, Santayana had a soft spot in his heart for religion, viewing faith traditions as indispensable despite their supernatural fictions, because they have the power to nurture the senses of piety, humility, and awe that humanity needs to keep its ego in check.

Santayana wrote that there is wisdom in cultivating "man's reverent attachment to the sources of his being and the steadying of his life by that attachment." Reason will not grow up until it integrates roles for faith, ethics, and other journeymen of the subjective realm to join science and logic on the quest for a relationship to the world that works.

By continually producing the most fitting response to life that we can muster, learning what we can from the effort, and carrying the most useful wisdom forward, *what is* and *what ought to be* will naturally and logically become more obvious parts of a larger whole.

A merger of faith, reason, and ethics will help our cultural systems find the state of metabolic balance they need—provided the elites who run our powerful institutions get on board with the call to meet global challenges and approach a more stable state of health and sustainability. This claim is not based on philosophical argument; it is a working hypothesis generated by an integrative clinical mind-set.

Application of an integrative clinical mind-set to questions traditionally taken up by scientists, philosophers, theologians, and ethicists yields not another argument shot full of holes, but instead a clinical hypothesis to be tested through actual experiment, or, failing that, thought experiment. As thought experiment then, a hypothesis:

Integrating faith, reason, and ethics into a coherent worldview, with support from a growing network of power-wielding elites near the centermost positions of the institutions that operate in our major cultures, will guide our social, political, economic, and environmental systems on a path to health and sustainability.

This hypothesis is testable. All that is required is a randomized, double-blinded, placebo-controlled trial involving a few thousand planets where a dominant species faces health and sustainability dilemmas similar to our own. What should we do in the meantime?

The revelations of religious history carry the flaws of the human beings who transmitted or edited them, but they also carry forward the crux of our highest aspirations and virtues. Literal truth may lie eternally beyond our reach; a culturally integrated wisdom will be our best guide for navigating reality and charting a course to global wellness.

Wisdom will be enriched by the partnership of faith, reason, and ethics; the integration of these ways of interpreting meaning can teach us to stand in awe of the mystery, subtlety, and complexity of being, yet also to accept responsibility and accountability for valuing and acting upon the relevant objective and subjective knowledge we have at hand.

A law of reason may look like a guillotine for a century or two, only to appear as a crochet hook later on because new information changes how the over-arching mystery casts its shadows. Our minds come to see that by using the hooks of intellect and emotion, weaving faith, reason, and ethics together can form a cultural mesh capable of withstanding the inevitable counter-offensives of the world's plunderers—and a banner of hope for those who would be stewards of the Earth.

Wisdom gathers ideas of theoretical, moral, and practical value, and knits them into an increasingly coherent bigger picture; it values the idea that human beings exist for a purpose, but accepts that human beings are not the final measure of such things.

We are in no position to state with absolute confidence what our purpose is—which is precisely why we need to keep listening and adapting to reality and to our interpretations of reality.

As bodymind wisdom evolves into the twenty-first century, it seems to be telling us that our job, both as individuals and as a species of intelligent life, is to discern as best we can what the mysterious force of creation wants us to be and to do.

From a clinical standpoint, it would appear at this stage in our evolution that what we are meant to be is humble, and what we are to do is become as fully integrated and ethically responsible as we can.

The map of how to get there is under our noses. Nature, in its patterns and processes of interdependence, continuously illustrates how self-organizing and integrating systems can become ever more functional parts within ever more robust, socially cooperative wholes. The better we pattern our cultural change policies on examples drawn from cells, organisms, and ecosystems, the more likely we are to stay on top as stewards in the Earth system game.

Looking at the Earth from twenty thousand miles away, imagine seven billion astoundingly complex products of creation and evolution trying to find their way on a big, blue planet. Pan back and see this same planet, teeming with life and meaning, joy and suffering, as a pale blue dot that is home to both the pride and the trash of the universe. Will we learn to seek wisdom together, to value health, integrate, and aim higher as one bodymind? Can we transform ourselves?

As Andrew Bourke notes in his conclusion to *The Principles of Social Evolution*, there are open questions concerning the mechanisms of the major evolutionary transitions. One of these questions is:

> Which of the following affects social traits more strongly: variation in relatedness or variation in the non-genetic parameters in Hamilton's Rule?

You may think this is a boring question, so let's translate it. In the major evolutionary transitions so far, genetic relatedness predicts a higher tendency toward cooperation. In the next major evolutionary transition in the Earth system, the one that humanity can lead, it is unclear whether our species as a whole shares enough genetic relatedness to promote the level of social cooperation that major transitions seem to require. Thus, we are starring in an evolutionary cliffhanger!

What gives us hope is our knowledge that human minds, and the cultures that have arisen from the collective actions of such minds, are in possession of free will and moral sense. With these newly evolved features, the species may have at its disposal a means by which to free itself from the strict familial limits of genetic relatedness as a condition for social cooperation.

Although every member of our species shares most of the genes held by every other member, that fact doesn't help us feel closely related. Cultural differences get in the way. Yet we are all directly related, not just to the first eukaryote to make the multi-celled transition, but also through our shared connection to a gradual process of organization and integration that began 13.7 billion years ago.

For most of this time, evolution was a random process of natural selection. But the random process of natural selection could well have become nonrandom at the point where free-willed, morally sensitive creatures with technological sophistication entered the narrative.

That is, natural evolution has all the appearance of a random selection process, until now, when the idea of convergence toward social cooperation as a survival strategy looms large in the auditorium of science. In the back of the room stands religion, straining to hear and make sense of a soul-changing idea: nature seems to be heading toward higher and higher levels of functional integration as if fulfilling some kind of purpose that is ours to discern—a purpose that may have been put into motion by a Maker, and in any event seems to align with essential teachings found in the sacred texts of most religions, and that also aligns with the kind of mental, social, and institutional shifts that health and sustainability will require of us.

The path to the health and sustainability of living systems leads also in the direction of human flourishing because it insists upon a major evolutionary transition that can only emerge from a cross-cultural emphasis on social cooperation. This means that God *and* evolution, our most valued sacred and secular worldviews, are confronting us to do the same thing that they can do: cooperate. The evolutionary path to health and sustainability eerily and unexpectedly converges with the proverbial path to heaven on Earth. What happens next depends on the choices that we, as human beings, and we, as a species, make in the twenty-first century.

One Faith to Bind Them All and in the Darkness Guide Them

◇◇◇◇◇◇◇◇◇◇◇◇◇◇◇◇◇◇◇◇◇◇◇◇◇◇◇◇◇◇◇◇◇

Not counting orcs and sociopaths whose brains fail to develop moral circuits, ninety-nine percent of us share the sense that it is our responsibility to become the kind of person who adheres to basic social conventions about the right and the good.

In his book *The Responsible Self*, theological ethicist H. Richard Niebuhr (1894–1962) argues that the proper first question of ethics is not, "What is right?" or "What is good?" but rather, "What is going on?" It makes sense that the first question of ethics should be identical to the first question physicians ask when they approach someone with the intent to heal. Like medicine, ethics depends on robust description of what's going on before prescribing any solutions; their jobs are to figure out what to do with the evidence at hand, medicine with a purpose to heal, and ethics with a purpose to promote the right and the good in ways that are wise and virtuous.

"What's going on?" is really the proper first question in any attempt to make sense of the world and our place in it. And the answer that precedes all others is this: a mysterious creative force acted in such a way as to allow us to happen, and now we are in the position of deciding how we ought to respond, both as individuals and as a collective species of being.

A former student of Niebuhr's, theological ethicist James M. Gustafson (1928–2003), echoed the idea that ethical questions about the right and the good are logically preceded by the context of what's going on in natural creation. The foremost task of theological ethics is to discern proper ways of responding to the idea that God created nature, and that we therefore must face the task of discerning God's plan for wisdom and virtue with courage in an ever-evolving and mysterious universe.

Gustafson urged careful thinkers to bring all forms of reliable knowledge to this task. This meant that religious beliefs had to be reconciled with the facts and theories of science.

A former student of Gustafson's, theological ethicist Stephen J. Pope was influenced by his mentor's position on the relationship between theology, ethics, and scientific knowledge. In his book *Human Evolution and Christian Ethics*, Pope addresses Gustafson's point when he writes that science provides an "epistemologically optimal vantage point from which to understand the world in which we live" and that as a "matter of intellectual integrity one cannot be confined to Christian accounts of truth."

What Gustafson and Pope endorse is a turning away from sole reliance on Christian accounts of the truth when those "truths" contradict the facts and laws of science, such as the growing mountain of physical evidence for evolution by natural selection. This turn in philosophical theology underpins the turn to a theistic evolutionary worldview.

Should more churches and religious leaders adopt this view, they would help to build a more functional portal between faith and reason, boosting prospects that cooperative faith- and science-based efforts can bolster the health and sustainability of the Earth system.

A clinical approach to problem solving loses its own functional integrity when it submits itself to dogmatic beliefs that cannot be reconciled with scientific knowledge about how nature works. The same can be said for attempts by dogmatic religious subcultures that seek to impose their particular beliefs and behaviors on the culture at large.

But let's be clear about what constitutes scientific knowledge. The theory of evolution is supported by rock-solid fossil evidence that translates into highly trustworthy scientific knowledge. This does not mean that we know everything we'd like to know about evolution. With every advance in evolutionary science, new questions pop up. But as this cycle moves forward, our knowledge about the genetic, biological, psychological, and social features of evolution become more reliable at increasingly granular levels.

What about medical science, the field charged with creating practical applications that physicians might use to get better results for their patients? Here, sorting the true and useful from true but useless information is a different story.

Most interpretations of scientific data are varnished with several coats of bias. One coat comes from researchers and publishers who are naturally invested in collecting and presenting novel findings that are statistically significant and thus able to draw more than the usual amount of attention. This is called *publication bias*.

A second coat comes from researchers who unconsciously filter their data during the act of measurement, choosing what gets documented. This is called *selective reporting*, a well-documented, widespread phenomenon that indicates a tendency for scientists to see in their data whatever it is they already want to believe.

A third coat comes from companies or investors with a financial stake in how scientific research gets interpreted. They hire experts to tweak the stats, ghostwriters to present the data in a light that best favors their product or idea, and industry thought leaders to hammer the message home with academic credibility. This is called *market bias* and it is powered by profit motive. The higher the stakes, the more tempting it gets to shoehorn the data to fit a message that willfully misleads the public—otherwise known as *fraud*. Literally dozens of other biases can undermine the validity or reliability of published scientific research.

So to be more precise, the optimal vantage point for knowledge is not science but *unvarnished* science—a more rarely seen bird that can be hard to spot in the wilds of medical research publishing.

John Ioannidis, MD, DSc, is an epidemiologist at Stanford University Medical School. His 2005 Public Library of Science article, "Why Most Published Research Findings Are False," is one of the most cited medical papers in recent history. This paper mathematically proves why we should expect over 80 percent of published research findings in medicine to be false.

Let's be candid. Most scientific research leads us somewhere other than truth. Even the highest-quality research at best leads us *toward* the truth, but not all the way to it. As Konrad Lorenz

(1903–1989), a pioneer in the science of animal behavior, once said, "Truth in science can be defined as the working hypothesis best suited to open the way to the next better one."

Scientific method gives us a way to create ever more valid and reliable truth approximations about reality without ever getting us to absolute truth. What good science creates is an asymptotic curve that ever more closely approaches truthiness about reality and being.

The most that science can offer us is a collection of increasingly valid and reliable truth approximations about what is really going on—but what a stupendously practical offering it is. Science has worked wonders for humankind and will continue to do so. While science remains the optimal vantage point from which to view the workings of the world, biases hidden under coats of varnish should compel us to interpret published research findings with caution. Planetary medical doctors, regular physicians, and their patients are in the market for medical wisdom; relatively true but useless findings do not serve their needs.

Like bad religion, bad science will lead us down paths we'll wish we hadn't taken. And while good science is our ally, it alone cannot lead us to health and sustainability. The Royal Society, the august assembly whose membership once included Sir Isaac Newton himself, acknowledges that if we are to meet the grand challenges of health and sustainability, the hard sciences must build gateways to the softer sciences and even to nontraditional sources of knowledge. These less-than-traditional sources of knowledge include insights that are grounded in faith, intuition, creativity, and all the arts of the Humanities.

From a clinical standpoint, the value of an evidence claim is not determined by its testability, but by its ability to interpret facts in ways that promote meaning and hope that can support health and sustainability. To the integrative clinical mind, theological perspective can be a source of high-value insight for those aiming to solve the problems now facing the living systems of the world.

Human ways of knowing should be allowed to draw from physics and from metaphysics, as they are both part of the same whole. What's needed to transform knowledge into wisdom is a commitment to intellectual integrity—an honest rationality that supervises the ongoing construction of a fully integrated description of what's going on in the Earth system.

Gustafson's position is that while science provides an optimal vantage point for making objective sense of the world, subjective theological perspective has the potential to help us make even more sense of it.

In Volume One of *Ethics from a Theocentric Perspective*, Gustafson argues that the most basic task of believers is to discern, as best they can, what a Creator would want believers to be and to do. He points out that whether or not you believe in God, all your attempts to discern the best understandings of the right and the good exist within the context of a creative force that brought the universe into being, and that it is wise to consider that this force may have been put into motion by God.

Gustafson suggests that trying to discern a system of ethics without acknowledging that the context for nature includes the possibility of God is like trying to feed oneself without a head. Just as theologians should take into account scientific facts, scientists should weigh their facts in the light of the possibility that we are part of God's creation.

What likely makes belief difficult for the majority of scientists is the way religious traditions contradict themselves—let alone how they insist natural history included supernatural events or historical interpretations that justify one religious tradition more than another.

Do you believe in God? If so, is yours a mysterious God, or does your belief include a more detailed description of what God is like? For example, did your God:

A. Make a covenant with a chosen people and reveal the Ten Commandments to Moses?

B. Make a new covenant with the world by sending His son Jesus Christ to show you the way and the life and be your savior?

C. Restore an uncorrupted faith in the One True God through Muhammad (God praise his name), his last and greatest prophet?

D. All of the above.

E. None of the above.

To hold any of the above beliefs about God may be a perfectly healthy practice for you, your family, your congregation, or your community. So why must these closely related *One True God* faith traditions compete like bitter rivals?

Jews, Christians, and Muslims share a common origin in history. Each of their traditions stems from one of the Abrahamic religions. Though they seem to agree on the Golden Rule and other fundamental tenets of faith and the spiritual life, they can't seem to agree on the mundane rules of each faith without creating the kind of friction that results in spiritual blisters. Perhaps they rightly fear that their distinct rules and rituals are being exploited for reasons having to do with geopolitics, economics, and the defense of institutional power. Such manipulations reinforce trivial differences and obscure the essence of what these great faith traditions have in common, not least of which is the ethic to *love thy neighbor*.

From a planetary medicine standpoint, this is a form of metabolic dysfunction. While each of the Abrahamic traditions is rich with meaning and inspiration, the children of Isaac and Ishmael have not been able to form a higher-order level of functional integrity from which to serve what is, in the end, the same One True God of their beliefs.

This may change in part with the help of people like Harvard professor and negotiation expert William Ury, who spearheaded an innovative cultural integration program called *Abraham's Path, or Masar Ibrahim al Khalil*. As a form of cultural tourism, Ury and his collaborators developed a walking route that follows the footsteps of Abraham (Ibrahim) through the Middle East. The national trails wind through Turkey, Syria, Jordan, Palestine, and Israel. Extensions into Iraq are planned.

This initiative is a way of reconnecting the family of Abraham step by step. In this way it may win hearts and minds to the idea that Muslims, Christians, and Jews can again peacefully coexist, even collaborate, on projects that branch into directions where social cooperation and cultural integration are possible. This initiative is noteworthy in that it creates a physical path that symbolizes what the infrastructure of health and sustainability can look like in the future.

Assume for a moment that the Abrahamic monotheists of the Earth system had achieved a high level of harmony and effectiveness in serving their God, and that you were part of a secret contingent from another solar system whose task was to reverse-engineer how they did it. What would your report conclude? How did humanity pull off the Earth system's first *willed* major transition in the history of social evolution? Imagine this excerpt from such a report:

WILLED EVOLUTIONARY TRANSITIONS:

THE CASE OF *HOMO SAPIENS* AND PLANET EARTH

ALPHA QUADRANT SUSTAINABILITY COMMISSION

TRANSITION DYNAMICS

The AQ Surveillance team hacked into world libraries, broadcast archives, and social networks to develop a narrative history of the dominant species, *Homo sapiens.*

Over a mere two hundred thousand years, this species went from inventing primitive tools to developing social institutions and scientific technologies that, combined with rapid population growth, created a series of energy, cultural, economic, political, environmental, and health crises. During the prior four billion years, all evolutionary transitions had been gene-centric. Species leaders recognized that a transition to health and sustainability was needed, that a genetically paced transition would be too slow, and therefore that the transition would have to be driven by a conscious choice to organize and integrate diverse cultures toward healthy and sustainable changes.

A momentum-building dynamic took hold when moderates within their three primary monotheistic faith traditions facilitated new channels of cross-cultural communication, creating conditions for social trust and cooperation among groups previously fragmented by contrary belief systems.

Among their Jewish, Christian, and Muslim traditions for worshipping the One True God, evidence of mutual respect and desire for collaboration unfolded as the fundamentalists within each tradition established new ways of connecting and seeing what values they had in common. There emerged a shared sense of purpose strong enough to override fears about their religious differences. Variations in rules and rituals that for centuries had been seen as threats came to be seen as innocent and welcome forms of cultural diversity—alternate ways of adorning the main beam of their beliefs.

The monotheists formed agreeable connections with Hindus and with followers of Confucius, Buddha, and other sources of spiritual wisdom, including secular humanism, because they recognized how these connections strengthened humanity's spiritual core and brought ethics more to the fore in personal and public life—goals shared by all religious traditions.

This new spiritual coalition also gave rise to a broadly based change in consumer mentality that involved using group-purchasing models to coerce businesses into finding innovative ways to honor consumer preferences for business transparency, for a cleaner, more stable environment, for children's rights to nourishment, emotional care, and education, and for fair opportunities to obtain work and to lead dignified lives.

This consumer force also broke some of the control that political actors had maintained over cash flow dynamics within market sectors and election campaigns. Elected officials had little choice but to cater to a voting citizenry empowered by their coordinated purchasing power. A coalition of consumers and all but the largest employers forced the most powerful corporations to rethink their lobbying strategies and tactics. They were supported by the medical profession, which gradually de-fragmented itself and led a rolling drumbeat for health and sustainability. Using social network applications, this unlikely association of businesses, consumers, and medicine also managed to bring full transparency to business and politics.

When the new wave of social cooperation among the world's consumers joined the new wave of affiliated religious and secular wisdom traditions, there emerged a new force for change. Not only was there a quicker pace for the translation of clean scientific findings into practical uses, but also a more coherent cultural framework for fitting scientific findings into health and sustainability solutions for the Earth system as a whole.

In sum, never before in the history of willed evolutionary transitions has the AQ witnessed such a dramatic last-minute comeback story. The experience of *Homo sapiens'* willed transformation of the Earth system serves as an AQ object lesson on methods for moving the transitional setting from gene-driven to gene-and-culture-driven transformations.

An online coalition of conscientious citizen-consumers is not a pie-in-the-sky concept. Social networks have the ability to connect hundreds of millions of households. Facebook alone has over eight hundred million users, a number that is expected to continue to climb with Twitter and Google+ on their heels. At least 15 percent of the world's population is already within a few clicks of becoming a social network of consumers aimed at using their purchasing power to help drive health and sustainability initiatives.

Such a movement might exemplify what Chris Anderson the British media mogul calls *crowd accelerated innovation*, and what Chris Anderson the editor of *Wired* magazine calls *the long tail*.

Crowd accelerated innovation is possible when online content shows people how to excel at something they are passionate about. Video typically packs more punch, but other forms of content can accelerate imitation and innovation as well.

For the health and sustainability movement, the key is to attract a large enough crowd using content that combines technical or artistic excellence with innovation. In this way the coalition that will blaze trails to wellness and sustainable living will continue to grow. The larger the crowd, the more likely it is to contain the observers, skeptics, cheerleaders, trend-spotters, fact-checkers, and super-spreaders needed to fuel a cycle of rapid learning that leads to even more innovation.

The long tail is formed when a broad range of consumers support markets for lower-popularity items. Surprisingly, a broad range of low-popularity items tends to create more market share than a narrow range of highly popular items. Many businesses can expand their market share by catering to these smaller markets, but the long tail has another valuable property: it brings diversity to the market for meaningful new ideas that might lead to values worth sharing.

Here's the rub: the tipping point for a consumer-driven health and sustainability coalition is likely to occur only when health and sustainability becomes the most appropriate choice among market options for a given product or service. In a sagging economy, will consumers be willing to pay a premium for products and services that promote health and sustainability goals? How can we balance the tradeoffs between the consumer's interests in finding a good bargain with our species' interest in bargaining for its own sustainability?

Get your thinking caps on. At *onebodymind.com* we see the need for a coherent synthesis of ideas to help our species address its religious, political, economic, and environmental conundrums. We're searching for a rich vein of cognitive surplus to help develop traction toward a healthier, more sustainable Earth system. We do this so we can, you know, say we did it—to set a good example for the alpha quadrant, help our Maker win that bet with the devil, or maybe even create conditions that will sponsor human flourishing for generations to come.

We're looking for ideas and innovations that can help build the spiritual solidarity we'll need to become better stewards of the part of creation that's within our sphere of influence.

The more we hitch our goals to health and wellness, the more likely it is that we'll become accountable to something more loosely defined that remains nonetheless far greater than ourselves, to honor freedom and the responsibilities that come with it, and to take charge of creating a more fitting response to our shared condition.

We need to outgrow our tendency to assume that we know what's really going on in the cosmic story. Some go so far as to conclude that creation happened *in order* for something like us to happen. In the field of cosmology this is known as the strong form of the *anthropic principle*: the idea that the universe knew we were coming, that the mysterious creative force combined energy, substance, and time in such a way that we *had to happen*. If this is true—and perhaps it is—we still have no warrant to conclude that the story somehow hinges on us. We may amount to nothing more than a temporary presence on a pale blue dot in a spiral arm of the Milky Way, one of five hundred billion galaxies in the universe we call home. But is that any reason to do anything but our best to make our part of the story a tale of inspiration and purposes fulfilled?

The weaker form of the anthropic principle holds that the physical constants so far discovered make it extremely unlikely that the appearance of humanity occurred by chance. That is, if the universe didn't know we were coming, yet here we are, it was an extremely lucky roll of the dice. Is that any reason to do anything but our best to make our part of the story a tale of inspiration and purposes fulfilled?

The strong and weak forms of the anthropic principle leave us with two options: either the universe came factory-installed with a purpose, or it evolved without purpose until now, when we have the opportunity to lead evolution in the direction of social cooperation, which just so happens to point in the direction of *love thy neighbor*.

Rob Bell is the founder and lead pastor of Mars Hill Bible Church in Grand Rapids, Michigan. As of March 2011, Sunday attendance runs between eight thousand and ten thousand people. Bell is a creative person who uses his talents to reframe orthodox Christian doctrine with questions, leaving his followers to puzzle over the answers without ever straying too far from an orthodox Christian narrative of history.

In his book *Love Wins*, Bell takes up the subjects of heaven and hell. First is heaven. He writes:

> For all of the questions and confusion about just what heaven is and who will be there, the one thing that appears to unite all of the speculation is the generally agreed-upon notion that heaven is, obviously, *somewhere else*.

Then, on the promises made by the prophets concerning life in the age to come:

First, they spoke about "all the nations." That's *everybody*. That's all those different skin colors, languages, dialects, and accents; all those kinds of food and music; all those customs, habits, patterns, clothing, traditions, and ways of celebrating—multi-ethnic, multi-sensory, multi-everything...A racist would be miserable in the world to come.

On what the faithful thought in Jesus' first-century world, and the implications for today, and perhaps for an age of health and sustainability to come, Bell writes:

They did not talk about a future life *somewhere else*, because they anticipated a coming day when the world would be restored, renewed, and redeemed and there would be peace on earth.

Jesus teaches us to pursue the life of heaven now...anticipating the day when heaven and earth are one. Honest business, redemptive art, honorable law, sustainable living, medicine, education, making a home, tending a garden—they're all sacred tasks to be done in partnership with God now because they will all go on in the age to come.

If you believe that you're going to leave and evacuate to *somewhere else*, then why do anything about this world?

This notion of heaven comforts, but it also confronts by urging us to transform our ways, to drop our preconceived notions of *us* versus *them*, of the *saved* versus *the damned*. Bell lays out multiple-choice answers:

So how do I answer questions about heaven? How would I summarize all that Jesus teaches? There's heaven now, somewhere else. There's heaven here, sometime else. And then there's Jesus' invitation to heaven here and now, in this moment, in this place.

And then there is hell, a prison where the damned have been sentenced to endless "fury, wrath, fire, torment, judgment, eternal agony, endless anguish." How does this square with the God of healing, redemption, and love? Bell concludes:

> We need a loaded, volatile, adequately violent, dramatic, serious word to describe the very real consequences we experience when we reject the good and true and beautiful life that God has for us. We need a word that refers to the big, wide, terrible evil that comes from the secrets hidden deep within our hearts all the way to the massive, society-wide collapse and chaos that comes when we fail to live in God's world, God's way.

Though Bell never endorses the idea of *universal reconciliation*—the notion that *all* souls will mercifully be reconciled with God, not just the souls supposedly saved by having sufficiently correct beliefs—he leaves the door to universal reconciliation open enough to be charged as a heretic by figures representing reformed Protestant churches.

While *heretic* derives from the Greek word for "free to choose," the word is used to put a target on the accused because the word carries with it a sense of shame for having freely chosen to deviate from an established doctrine. Religious denominations have their own doctrines, but so do political, academic, and professional subcultures; shame can systematically be used to deter divergent thinking by members of any flock.

The Mars Hill Bible Church's statement on narrative theology is nowhere near heretical. A functional medicine doctor billing insurance for the time needed to generate a detailed health narrative for a patient? *That's* heretical.

From a somewhat heretical clinical standpoint, then, believers should feel safer to reconcile the historical particulars of their religious narratives to the Big History of evolution, because any policy that helps humanity become a flock unified on the factual basics represents a step toward health and sustainability. I'm not out to topple church doctrines—I'm in search of a clinical path that can lead us in the direction of transforming our self-imposed hellish realities into something a bit more heavenly.

Doctrines found blocking this path, whether they arise from religious, political, academic, professional, or other sources, should be considered pathological; they stand in the way of the greater functional integrity our species will need if we are to approach that destination where our healthiest doctrines about love, wisdom, and virtue seem already to be pointing: a healthy and sustainable Earth system marked by a human relationship to the world that works.

The institutions of science and technology cannot, by themselves, guide us to such a place. So, welcome aboard one and all. Work out your doctrinal squabbles when the storm settles. Right now, it's all hands on deck.

The visionary physician Albert Schweitzer (1875–1965) felt that we are called to the role of bringing the highest possible wisdom and compassion into the relationships that fall within our sphere of reach, and that the world would become a healthier place if we did our best to respond to this call. Before this noble sentiment are strewn mighty obstacles.

Among them is our instinctual, anxiety-driven need to put our own interests ahead of the interests of other people and things, and ahead of the interests of the greater whole. This angst drives us to accept short-term gain even when it means long-term pain for ourselves and for others including our own descendants.

Being biological creatures with reptilian brain parts, it's only natural for us to interpret data and seek ways to reduce our anxieties and improve our standing in the world. But when, to control our anxieties, we make ourselves the measure of all things, we lose humility and risk our ability to join faith, reason, and ethics in a more powerful quest for a healthier future.

When we achieve self-certainty about what heaven is and who will be there, or what hell is and who shall suffer eternal damnation and why, we disrupt the metabolism of social cooperation. Switch two letters in the word *united* and you get *untied*; the words are like a protein that can fold two ways—where one conformation conveys a meaning virtually opposite to the other. From a systems biology point of view, we are in need of meanings that can fold as needed to underwrite the functional integrity required by health and sustainability. We need to untie the knots of literalism and premature certainty to relieve the spasms that prevent us from creating a cultural physiology that can sustain unity in diversity.

From the standpoint of a planetary medicine doctor, it would be good practice to emphasize that the path to humility begins with the fact that an entire cosmos of interdependent relationships was created *not by us*. If you want to be in charge of the laws, create your own universe. Otherwise be humble and listen, as your true condition is unknown by you. Yet if your cultures can build trust and maintain an open collective mind, your true condition will grow more discernable, and your future more manageable, in due course.

If you're a secular humanist, be in charge of making ethics matter. If you are a religious or spiritual person, let your core values guide your actions but question your intolerance for people who have similar core values but who dare to express them in their own way. It is enough to abhor evil and to work to diminish its presence. As for the rest, we are in it together. Promote health and wellness within your sphere of influence and you help lay the groundwork for a willed evolutionary transition toward something away from existential hell and closer to spiritual heaven on Earth.

The World's Most Epic Game

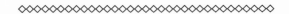

Imagine we could perform a randomized controlled planetary trial in which various planetary dominant species confronted with health and sustainability problems were randomly sorted into one of two groups:

1. An experimental group that consults planetary doctors who provide a cultural change regimen that calls for the integration of faith, reason, and ethics.

2. A control group that consults planetary doctors who provide "usual care" (recommendations on the use of summits, sanctions, treaties, bailouts, and other procedures as needed).

Here's the hypothesis: the living systems on the planets of the experimental group would become healthier than the living systems on the planets of the control group, and, barring unexpected catastrophes, they would remain that way over the period of the study and beyond.

Say the study got done. Researchers enrolled one hundred planets whose living systems were dominated by a species struggling to survive in the industrialized, politicized, trade-imbalanced, culturally splintered bed they'd made for themselves.

These planets were randomized into two groups of fifty each. The species in the study group agreed to commit to a cultural change that would have them unite around a powerful but simple faith; the species in the control group took advice on how to manage symptoms using various conflict resolution methods but essentially did whatever they felt like doing. The living systems on each planet were then monitored for four hundred years for signs of health gains or declines.

If the evidence supports the hypothesis, then the living systems on "unified faith" planets would have fared better on average, as documented by their comparative progress in managing the one thousand markers of ecosystem and cultural health followed in the study. These markers ranged from quality of education, renewable energy sources, social trust, and corruption levels to hundreds of markers of pollution and mismanagement affecting air, water, land, minerals, crops, habitats, and ecosystems. What kind of results would such an experiment find?

Imagine that a team of galactic archeologists found a capsule in the subsoil of a once habitable rocky planet in the gamma quadrant. In the capsule, they found Buzz Lightyear holding a jump drive in his outstretched hand, The drive contained all the raw data of the study described above. After analyzing it, they distilled the meaning of the data down to three sentences:

Health improvements showed up within thirty years, and rose for an average of 150 years, with achieved gains maintained for the duration of the study. The most accurate predictor of a flourishing dominant species and of planetary system sustainability was the rate at which the infants of the dominants formed secure attachments to their parents. When that rate exceeded 50%, social trust levels climbed above 75%, and cultures entered a gradual period of transformation in which they changed from being destroyers to being good stewards of living systems.

What exactly happened on the *unified faith* planets to account for these results? What were the mechanics of change that led to healthier living systems? What alterations in the dominant species brought living systems into a more stable form of metabolic balance?

By uniting around a simple body of faith, did the dominant species up-regulate pathways that participate in the synthesis of health and wellness within multiple spheres of influence?

Did social cooperation and market adaptations help turn these troubled, dominant life forms into stewards able to balance the need for development with the needs of the environment? By some kind of personal or social discipline did they develop cross-cultural bonds that led to better translations of the wisdom and compassion found within their respective traditions? Did all of this follow a focused effort to rear securely attached children, placing the children in better position to become emotionally balanced and socially responsible adults?

Thankfully, the drive also contained an executive summary by the panel of planetary medicine doctors that reviewed the raw data, including interviews of the descendants of the participants in the study. Here's the abstract from their review:

UNIFIED FAITH AS A HEALTH AND SUSTAINABILITY STRATEGY

FOR ENDANGERED PLANETARY DOMINANTS: A REVIEW

Planetary Medical Collaborative Group

ABSTRACT

We reviewed raw data from the one hundred planets enrolled in the *Healing of Planetary Ecologies (HOPE) Study*.

What they did: We found that on the *unified faith* planets, the once-jeopardized dominant animals had several things thing in common:

1. Each had a heightened sense of urgency that current relationships to the other living systems on their planet were unsustainable.

2. Each caused to emerge a new cultural pathway that functioned like a self-regulating engine for social cooperation and ethical problem solving behavior.

3. Each species learned healthy ways to metabolize their cultural differences so they could organize around core spiritual ideals and principles of functional integrity.

How they did it: The most common way involved innovative use of a widely distributed, media-rich, broadband system of communication. Using this system, beings whose beliefs and behaviors were defined by cultures that had been closed off from one another were able to connect and share experience, knowledge, and values, creating history with each other that hadn't existed prior to development of a 24/7 social networking system that included language translations. It was as if the culturally distinct members of these species came to see themselves as being part of the same team, working together to win a game called "Fix the Planet," which they could only win by fixing themselves.

On the unified faith planets, fear-driven social networks lost market share. Corporations and nonprofits grew market shares by demonstrating their commitments to personal wellness, public health, stewardship, and other communal goals. Fraud and corruption grew scarcer as transparency and real-time whistle blowing became cultural norms. Not wanting to get caught or blamed, transgressors changed their behaviors. Cultural systems also defeated fraud and corruption with early detection methods and adaptive quick-response mechanisms.

Over time, groups sprouting up within these web-like communication systems developed increasingly productive tools for tracking and spurring progress, called apps. Apps sped innovations for sharing knowledge expertise and translating it into health and sustainability action. They tapped into the unrealized potential of social cooperation, ethical vision, and a shared mission pursued with the urgent optimism.

They built trust and developed the social capital needed to aim as one for solutions to common problems. Previously disconnected groups realized that their motives and expectations were more similar than different, especially when it came to issues of nutrition, exercise, stress reduction, happiness, dignity, work, liberty, safety nets, infrastructure, corporate and political transparency, fiscal conservancy, intelligent urban design, renewable energy, and the ecological balance of living systems. Most importantly, they realized the utter importance of parent-child bonding, personalized education, and of healthy emotional care during childhood.

As their cultures became better organized and integrated, their institutions evolved in ways that made their social systems as a whole more functional and sustainable. By de-fragmenting their cultures, they created conditions suitable to the evolution of a global culture focused on core values. The wisdom of the crowd functioned like a *de novo* gene-regulation system, except it was social behavior, not genes, being regulated.

As the freethinking individual members of these species came to see the benefits of collaborative problem solving, they leveraged their cognitive surplus and social connections into healthy and sustainable forms of cultural change. "Heresy" became known as "brainstorming." Loosely connected tribes, subcultures, and nations developed like an embryo into a greater whole with functional integrity of immense logical and thermodynamic depth. Once-divided communities gradually merged into what was, for lack of a better term, one bodymind.

Just as evolution appears to converge on similar solutions for eyesight, it may also converge on similar solutions for ethical vision, as such vision gives rise to the heroic habits our species will need to become capable of producing an epic evolutionary win.

We don't know if distant life forms have reached or passed through the *willed* social evolutionary transition stage yet. We can afford to wait for nature to select a randomly occurring human pro-ethics gene about as much as we can afford to wait for planetary medical doctors from outer space to arrive with genetically modified stem cell injections designed to make us cooperate with each other. The near-term health of living systems on Earth has come down to a match between the selfish gene and the selfless will, or at least a collective will with enough rational self-interest to quest for health and sustainability.

We must become a collection of ethical beings, but also a culturally ethical global society. The rub is that cultures do not change unless sufficient force for change is brought to bear. When push comes to shove, that force packs projectiles and explosives. The new force for cultural change needs to reach a global consensus about what health and sustainability is requiring of us, and do so without need for pushing and shoving.

Thus far, neither faith in God nor secular love of the good has lifted our species onto a solid track toward health and sustainability. Every time we're done imagining a better way to run the world we open the window to find reality still staring us in the face, red in tooth and claw.

Global warming somehow remains up for debate, even though we have already settled the fact that whatever the cause, the planet has a fever, and we may have only a handful or two of decades to go before water rises up somewhere between the waists and necks of the world's floodplain-dwellers.

The time for lollygagging on this issue is long gone, but it is hard for people to relate to a trend that slowly unfolds over decades. *New York Times* columnist Thomas Friedman avoids the term *global warming* because it makes people don blinders in a hurry. Better to use a term that folks can relate to because it is happening before their eyes. Friedman prefers to call it *global weirding*.

Elizabeth Kolbert writes for *The New Yorker* and has won multiple awards for her reporting on climate change. In "Storms Brewing" (published in June, 2011), she addressed the intense weather events that affected the United States and other parts of world over a series of months. Floods and super-tornadoes took a massive toll from the Great Plains to the East coast. Droughts and forest fires roasted the southwest as the National Oceanic and

Atmospheric Administration announced that the 2011 hurricane season would produce a sixty-five-percent chance of "above normal" activity, predicting three to six major hurricanes, which produce wind levels over 110 mile per hour and storm surges beyond eight feet of water.

Little did Americans know that the season's most damaging hurricane would spin up the Eastern seaboard from the Carolinas to the Canadian shore causing property damage amounting to billions of dollars. Buried in all this weather news, wrote Kolbert, "The chief economist for the International Energy Agency, in Paris, announced that, despite the economic slowdown, global CO_2 emissions last year rose by a record amount, to almost thirty-one billion metric tons."

There is no denying that the weather gets weirder as the climates gets warmer. Kolbert points out that weirdly intense weather is a dysfunction caused by the physics of global warming. She writes:

For decades, climate scientists have predicted that, as global temperatures rose, the side effects would include deeper droughts, more intense flooding, and more ferocious storms. The details of these forecasts are immensely complicated, but the underlying science is pretty simple. Warm air can hold more moisture. This means that there is greater evaporation. It also means that there is more water, and hence more energy, available to the system.

What we are seeing now is these predictions being borne out. If no particular flood or drought or storm can be directly attributed to climate change—there's always the possibility that any single event was just a random occurrence—the overall trend toward more extreme weather follows from the heating of the earth.

Kolbert described President Obama's visits to Tuscaloosa, Memphis, and Joplin, where he asked unanswerable questions about cruel twists of fate, offering comfort to the people in these towns as they mourned their catastrophic losses. She then held up the President's timid track record on global warming and made her closing argument:

> Now that the immediate crisis has passed, the President needs to stop asking the kind of questions that can't be answered and start addressing those that can. Obama knows—and, indeed, has stated as much—that if we continue along our present path we'll guarantee our children a much more dangerous future. Taking the steps that would reduce the risks of climate change is not going to be politically popular, which is why it is the President's obligation to press for them. It may be beyond our power to control the climate, but we can determine it. This is precisely what we are doing, whether we choose to acknowledge it or not.

Have we entered an age in which international disaster relief efforts must compete for help from a world grown numb with compassion fatigue? Will climate change policy be banished from consideration at the behest of partisan election tactics and Super Pac ruses? Will our species become an apathetic loser with no wit or will to succeed in a game that began over thirteen billion years ago and that now asks us to choose between a path to stewardship and a path to destruction?

Any well-schooled planetary medicine doctor would be shocked by the Earth's rapidly changing biomarkers of ecosystems in decline. A quick surface scan of the Earth reveals a telling lesion in the Western hemisphere. Zooming in on this lesion reveals it to be a giant, floating scab—a continent-sized raft of garbage adrift in the Pacific. The implication is clear: planet Earth's ecosystems have been widely infiltrated by an invasive industrial species.

Humanity is now the dominant force in the long-evolving history of sustainable earthly adaptations. What is unclear is whether the human relationship to the world has gone past the point of repair, or whether it is capable of making a health and sustainability comeback.

The vocal minority that likes to perpetuate doubt about global warming misses the point: even if the easy-bake oven effect we're experiencing is not of our own making, we're still going to get scorched. Whether the cause of global warming is humanity's appetite for growth and development or a natural swing in climate trends, we confront the same problem: heat. We're like the patient who's just been advised to quit smoking, drinking, and sitting around eating ultra-processed junk food, whose "note to self" reads, "Find a better doctor."

In medicine, coaxing people into adopting healthier lifestyles has been the perennial tough nut to crack. The system doesn't reward doctors for putting in the effort, but even if it did, the results would tend to disappoint, because behavioral change is such an uphill battle. Yet the essential problem of healthy behavior change may already be solved: make the task emotionally engaging and meaningful.

Adam Bosworth has been a senior manager at several tech firms, including Microsoft and Google, where he headed the recently deceased Google Health division. After leaving Google, he founded a startup called Keas (pronounced key´-us). The Keas team set out to use online technology to help people live healthier lives. They made early mistakes, but then they stumbled onto a concept known as the power of play.

When Keas launched its care plans in 2009, they bombed. People would sign up and disappear within a couple weeks. The theory that interpretation of health risks, followed by the outlining of healthy action steps, would be enough to prompt users to make healthy changes was flat-out wrong. So Keas rounded up some medical experts and assembled the best health information they could find, as a way to draw a steady stream of online participation. User metrics did not improve.

The keyword "health" is typed into over five billion Google searches every year. Health is a fairly complicated topic, yet health info-seekers are known for their short attention spans. They'll give you about 10 seconds to produce something of interest before they move on to the next site. If you're an online health educator trying to do justice to a complicated health topic, you're apt to succumb to the TLDR problem: "Too long, didn't read." Potential users are gone before they get to the sentence that says quick and easy solutions don't work.

Given the pressure on startups, Keas had one more chance to re-engineer their platform. In late 2010, they launched a game that included quizzes and awarded points for self-reported healthy changes in diet, exercise, and stress reduction. It worked. According to Keas, the key success factor was peer pressure brought to bear in a game-play format.

They rolled out the program to large employers through human resource professionals who were avid partners with the concept. Employees formed small teams in which each member would make three commitments, choosing from among 150 possible healthy lifestyle changes. The data showed that over 40% of users would post at least once a week for twelve weeks or more. Many of the posts revealed users who wanted to be challenged even more.

A new word, absent from most dictionaries, captures what's going on here. It's called *gamification*, or engaging the power of play in a way that rewards people for progress toward a meaningful task. The power boost comes from the kind of peer pressure that holds team members accountable to each other for their results.

Given a properly structured game, Keas' users did not feel pushed; they were pulled into changing their behaviors because they felt an emotionally powerful reward for doing the right thing. If a dopamine-enhanced sense of team purpose can animate the will to solve such a difficult behavioral change puzzle, could it help save the world?

In *Reality is Broken: Why Games Make Us Better and How They Can Change the World*, Jane McGonigal notes that by the time our device-enabled children reach 21 years of age, they will have spent 10,000 hours navigating computer games and social networks. That is roughly the same amount of time they spend in school between fifth and twelfth grade. It also corresponds to the 10,000 hours of practice that is needed for someone to turn a talent into a highly exceptional level of excellence, as argued by Malcom Gladwell in *Outliers: The Story of Success*.

Having studied what, exactly, these young gamers are getting good at with all this time spent online, McGonigal found that they get really good at bringing four heroic habits to any important and rewarding challenge: urgent optimism, a willingness to be part of a social fabric, blissful productivity, and a sense of epic meaning.

If we wanted to engineer the heroic habits we need to win the modern quest for health and sustainability, we couldn't do a better job than *World of Warcraft*—an online game that has amassed 5.93 million years' worth of problems solved for members of the virtual world known as Azeroth. As McGonigal points out, 5.93 million years ago our hominid ancestors were solving the problem of standing upright. What if the talent and drive of virtuoso gamers were turned toward real-world problems of sustainability? McGonigal tested this idea by turning several unsolved real-world problems into games whose puzzles *had better* get solved or else the world would self-destruct.

One of these games is called *Superstruct!* It begins with a press release announcing that a supercomputer, having analyzed over 70 petabytes of environmental, economic, and demographic data, cross-validated by ten different probabilistic models, had reset the survival horizon for *Homo sapiens* from "indefinite" to a mere twenty-three years. In response to this news, a "Global Extinction Awareness Program" identified five "super-threats" needing immediate action.

Superstruct became the world's first massively multiplayer game to use a virtual construct to forecast ways of solving real-world problems. By signing on to play, you automatically became a member of the dream team being assembled to save humanity from extinction. The game collected over 500 credibly creative ideas about how to manage environmental, economic, social, technological, and behavioral threats to human survival.

You may have seen the parody of World of Warcraft players so addicted to the game that they become pimply blobs that would relieve themselves in bedpans rather than leave their screens. Games this absorbing can pose real health dangers. Sleep cycles get disrupted, fat mass increases as muscles shrink, and wrist splints fail to contain the nerve damage caused by a million clicks. Heroic virtual habits don't amount to much if the real-world result turns you into Jabba the Hutt. A balanced life is essential to personal health, just as urgent optimism and a sense of mission are essential to social health and sustainability.

Keas' gamification of healthy lifestyle change may produce unreliable metrics because user changes are largely based on unverified self-reports. Still, they have found the key to getting people engaged in an important task as a team, demonstrating in a thorny health arena how the power of play could be a boon to human problem solving potential.

Foursquare and Yelp are two companies that exploit the power of play as they compete in the arena for geolocation check-in and selling services. Use their mobile apps to post comments from one of their business client locations (typically a bar or restaurant), and you can earn a badge or achieve a higher rank in their system. Flash your badge to a bartender and you may get a free drink or a basket of tortilla chips. In this game system you are playing a version of "You scratch my back, I'll scratch yours," where the win-win bargain has variable levels of pull on you. How much does a free drink or a higher rank mean to you? As the power of play gets exploited in more meaningful ways, we could see more emotionally intense levels of engagement in quests that dangle what McGonigal calls the promise of "epic wins"—victories that mean something on a real world stage.

We see geo-location check-in systems like *ushahidi.com* being used to recruit people to coordinating sites for disaster relief, protest rallies, and victory celebrations—a win-win social bargain where badges and bargains are not the issue. Engaging in this kind of social bargain could mean putting yourself at risk in a real world setting. Your cyber-world traffic history can come back to hurt you if, say, you're a rebel in Syria and the police confiscate your phone.

The power of play creates an opportunity to turn the heroic habits rewarded in virtual reality settings into heroic habits rewarded in the real world. For example, a company's sustainability ranking could become a mark of quality that includes support for a larger social purpose, which then can translate into increased market share for a range of products and services. Or someone who raised money to fund an African water project could win a free stay at a participating hotel or dinner for two at a participating restaurant. The possibilities are endless. A check-in service that motivates pub-crawling amounts to stressing one's liver to help local businesses. What will motivate social cooperation on a higher scale of value? Game designers must figure out how to reward courageous leadership and the sharing of problem solving advice or innovative ideas and methods for team–building.

To a planetary medicine doctor, gaming has intriguing potential to become a force able to inspire heroic deeds and transformative new approaches to group problem solving.

The work of Ijad Madisch, a Harvard-trained virologist and computer scientist, qualifies for the kind of transformational thinking taking place in the world of scientific collaboration and publication. Madisch founded ResearchGate, an open access website where scientists can network and share ideas and papers without the friction and delays found in the traditional routes to getting published. Described as a Facebook for scientists, *ResearchGate* uses "like" and "follow" buttons to track the contributions of its members, who can accumulate reputation points.

This is not the traditional method for conducting peer review, but in the closed, copyright-protected world of science journal publication, most of the peer review is done for free by volunteers, many of whom are drawn to the open system that Madisch and colleagues are building for the scientific community.

If I were to write a simplified model for using connectivity to promote learning, trust, social cooperation, heroism, and cultural change in the direction of health and sustainability that would fit on a napkin, it would look something like this:

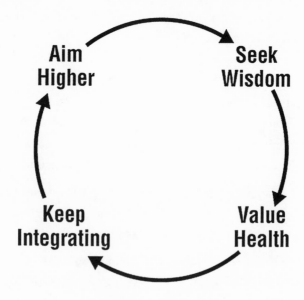

The same model could just as easily describe a gaming strategy for becoming good stewards of life and human welfare. The repeating loop puts an idealistic realism to the mission of health and sustainability in an open system of collaboration without borders; it is a rudimentary game plan for a real *World of Wellcraft*.

In their book, *The Innovator's Prescription*, Clayton Christensen, Jason Hwang, MD, and the late Jerome Grossman, MD (1940-2008), observe that the conventional approach to life sciences research and clinical problem solving rarely crosses boundaries between disciplines. This will change, and not just in the life sciences, because the innovative research and new solutions we're looking for are most likely to be found at the intersections where science, faith, culture, society, technology, and business meet.

For well over a century biology has advanced by means of the reductionistic method, whose goal is reduce whole systems into smaller parts whose mechanisms can be more readily studied and understood. Now enters integrative science using mathematical models to describe and predict how networks, both cellular and social, regulate parts at other levels. The next stage of expertise will focus on translating this knowledge into problem-solving wisdom. Research in the life and social sciences, aided by organizations like ResearchGate, will form new hubs for connectivity across disciplines, forming an infrastructure without walls that supports a more integrative approach to science.

We're building some of these intersections at *onebodymind.com*. With help from our micropublishing platform, *The One Bodymind Reader*, content contributors are getting published, gaining visibility, and sharing in the rewards. Our *Reader* places no limit on the kinds of insight and creativity it hopes to empower at this early stage in the quest for health and sustainability.

You can be a scientist or health industry expert looking to engage other experts. You can be a health advocate—someone with a wellness experience to share in matters relating to personal or social health. You can be a seeker—someone looking for answers or perspective on matters of health, self-care, or responsible stewardship. Seekers can move along crosswalks to see what experts are making of advocate stories and perspectives. Experts can peek in to see what kinds of questions are coming from seekers, and so on. Within this kind of ecosystem, our members will help transform the way we go about promoting health and self-care, finding clues and action plans to sustainability along the way.

A potentially transformative globalization process is underway. Whether it can lead us in the direction of health and sustainability is not yet clear, but there is a case to be made for optimism and for your participation.

Yes, economies are slumping, cultures are clashing, the environment is deteriorating, and political systems appear increasingly at a loss about how to lead us toward a future in which humanity and living systems can flourish together. But these realities cannot obscure the spirit of cooperation that wants to rise up and transform broken human systems into fully functional and sustainable engines of health and human dignity.

In the book *Edward R. Murrow's This I Believe*, Dan Gediman and John Gregory compile brief essays that were delivered by prominent Americans on Murrow's radio program in the 1950s. Several of the spoken deliveries can be found on the website *thisibelieve.org*, including this one by the luminous writer, educator, and conservationist of the American West, Wallace Stegner:

> It is terribly difficult to say honestly, without posing or faking, what one truly and fundamentally believes. Reticence or an itch to make public confession may distort or dramatize what is really there to be said, and public expressions of belief are so closely associated with inspirational activity, and in fact so often stem from someone's desire to buck up the downhearted

and raise the general morale, that belief becomes an evangeli-
cal matter.

In all honesty, what I believe is neither inspirational nor evan-
gelical. Passionate faith I am suspicious of because it hangs
witches and burns heretics, and generally I am more in sym-
pathy with the witches and heretics than with the sectarians
who hang and burn them. I fear immoderate zeal, Christian,
Moslem, Communist, or whatever, because it restricts the
range of human understanding and the wise reconciliation of
human differences, and creates an orthodoxy with a sword in
its hand.

I cannot say that I am even a sound Christian, though the code
of conduct to which I subscribe was preached more eloquently
by Jesus Christ than by any other. About God I simply do not
know; I don't think I can know.

However far I have missed achieving it, I know that modera-
tion is one of the virtues I most believe in. But I believe as
well in a whole catalogue of Christian and classical virtues:
in kindness and generosity, in steadfastness and courage and
much else. I believe further that good depends not on things
but on the use we make of things.

Everything potent, from human love to atomic energy, is dangerous; it produces ill about as readily as good; it becomes
good only through the control, the discipline, the wisdom
with which we use it. Much of this control is social—a thing
which laws and institutions and uniforms enforce—but much
of it must be personal and I do not see how we can evade the
obligation to take full responsibility for what we individually
do.

Our reward for self-control and the acceptance of private responsibility is not necessarily money or power. Self-respect and the respect of others are quite enough.

All this is to say that I believe in conscience, not as something implanted by divine act, but as something learned from infancy from the tradition and society, which has bred us. The outward forms of virtue will vary greatly from nation to nation; a Chinese scholar of the old school, or an Indian raised on the Vedas and the Bhagavad Gita, has a conscience that will differ from mine. But in the essential outlines of what constitutes human decency we vary amazingly little. The Chinese and the Indian know as well as I do what kindness is, what generosity is, what fortitude is. They can define justice quite as accurately. It is only when they and I are blinded by tribal and denominational narrowness that we insist upon our differences and can recognize goodness only in the robes of our own crowd.

Man is a great enough creature and a great enough enigma to deserve both our pride and our compassion, and engage our fullest sense of mystery. I shall certainly never do as much with my life as I want to, and I shall sometimes fail miserably to live up to my conscience, whose word I do not distrust even when I can't obey it.

But I am terribly glad to be alive; and when I have wit enough to think about it, terribly proud to be a man and an American, with all the rights and privileges that those words connote; and most of all I am humble before the responsibilities that are also mine. For no right comes without a responsibility, and being born luckier than most of the world's millions, I am also born more obligated.

Around the world more people are able to look past religious and political differences to see the common values and sentiments that lay at the core of human decision-making and behavior. Should our superficial differences stand in the way of the social cooperation we'll need to meet our key global challenges?

In the twenty-first century, the quest for global health and sustainability will require massive levels of cognitive surplus and cross-cultural collaboration. Here, in no particular order, is a gamer's short to-do list:

1. *Raise* the international standard of living and find ways to feed the next two billion human beings, most of who will be born into poverty.

2. *Grow* our economies in sustainable ways that reduce the gap between rich and poor.

3. *Regulate* capital flow just enough to prevent regional or global market collapses.

4. *Maintain* fiscal gaps in key national economies within a stable range.

5. *Increase* honesty and transparency in government, business, the professions, and the media.

6. *Detect*, condemn, punish, and prevent corruption.

7. *Restrain* our appetites for fossil fuels, while transitioning to clean energy sources and detoxifying our ecosystems.

8. *Mitigate* the effects of increasing carbon emissions.

9. *Prevent* soil erosion, loss of biodiversity, loss of wild habitat, and the over-harvesting of species.

10. *Reverse* ocean acidification.

11. *Counteract* growth in the Great Pacific Garbage Patch and its effluent sludge.

12. *Lower demand* for non-biodegradable, disposable plastics.

13. *Inhibit* cultural intolerance that leads to militant extremism.

14. *Block* nuclear proliferation and terrorist access to weapons of mass destruction.

15. *Avoid* the forms of malnutrition caused by hunger and by an excess of junk calories.

16. *Reduce* the spread of HIV/AIDS, tuberculosis, malaria, dysentery, and other communicable diseases by improving public health and increasing access to clean water.

17. *Develop* systems to effectively manage a global wave of age-related chronic illness.

18. *Help* all nations prepare for and recover from natural disasters and pandemics.

19. *Improve* our ability to empower children in ways that will help them achieve their fullest potential as adults.

20. *Inspire* social cooperation toward solutions to health and sustainability problems.

Imagine asking for a global show of hands in response to the question, "Who wants to step up and be part of team that tries to tackle these twenty issues?" How many hands would go up? Probably a tiny percentage; it sounds like a lot of hard work. Then imagine a show of hands in response to this question: "Who wants to help determine the reward structure needed to assemble a team to tackle these twenty issues?" We might witness a more enthusiastic response.

The reward structure would not simply boil down to the old saw that time is money, because not all rewards are external. Prestige, self-respect, learning new skills, and being part of a collaborative effort to tackle an epic mission count for something too. As Clay Shirky notes in *Cognitive Surplus*, the original sense of the word "amateur" referred to someone who does something for the love of it. Amateurs are welcome on the quest for health and sustainability. A willingness to learn and a passion for solving problems will count as much, if not more, than a list of credentials.

What will this quest look like? At present, it looks like a self-organizing but still poorly integrated range of efforts around the globe whose purpose is to advance health and sustainability. Many of the groups involved are well established and highly accomplished. They use distinct strategies for engaging the public, the academic community, governments, and the private sector. Four examples are discussed below.

The *United Nations* and two-dozen other international organizations set out to achieve a set of *Millennium Development Goals* by 2015. In 2010, these groups issued a progress report. While there are many signs of positive change, most of the hill is left to climb. The collaborators committed to marshaling additional support to help achieve their goals by 2015. The Millennium Development Goals website offers twenty easy ways to get involved. What started as a widespread plea for support from large world governments evolved into a user-friendly online platform that invites individuals to lend their support to the mission in a way that best suits their ability to give. What started as a top-down model has become a hybrid of top-down and bottom-up.

The *Earth System Science Partnership* has issued challenges for achieving earth system sustainability by carefully coordinating research that can help improve our forecasting models, discover ways to make cultural change less disruptive and more manageable, and encourage the social and technological innovations that will smooth the way through a required sequence of behavioral and cultural transitions. This affiliation of scientific research organizations from France, Sweden, Switzerland, and the Netherlands put together an insightful overview of the tasks that we will have to face as a species if we want to avert serious metabolic disruptions in the Earth system. They represent a top-down model with the potential to interact more with the public at large.

The *Grand Challenges in Global Health* is a coalition of partners including the Bill and Melinda Gates Foundation, the Foundation for the National Institutes of Health, the Canadian Institutes of Health Research, and the Wellcome Trust. They are focusing funds and skills on removing practical obstacles to disease prevention and treatment. This effort draws on the resources of the coalition partners to fund grants for research and demonstration projects. Their top-down strategy of relying on leading professionals in a range of academic fields was a conscious choice. Involving amateurs in what is fundamentally a grant-making institution could be counter-productive.

LAUNCH is an example of systematically managed innovation aimed at solutions to sustainability problems. It can be found at *Launch.org*. Their tag line is "collective genius for a better world." This novel group—NASA (National Aeronautics and Space Administration), USAID (United States Agency for International Development), the Department of State, and Nike—offers a new model for coordinating sustainability ideas and initiatives on a global scale. Their website describes their methods and leadership:

> NASA, USAID, and Nike joined together to form LAUNCH in an effort to identify, showcase and support innovative approaches to global challenges through a series of forums. LAUNCH searches for visionaries, whose world-class ideas, technologies or programs show great promise for making tangible impacts on society. At the heart of this effort is the LAUNCH Council—a diverse and collaborative world-class body of entrepreneurs, venture capitalists, scientists, engineers, and leaders in government, media, and business who will help guide these innovations forward. The Council is a deep and varied group of peers—each accomplished and visionary in their own work—each contributing to the cumulative power and wisdom of the LAUNCH network.

Here is a model that relies on a broad range of professional-level expertise and experience, but whose process sifts through creative, often disruptive ideas that have the potential to solve real world problems. LAUNCH currently focuses on issues related to water, health, air, and energy, but its model can extend to the full agenda of sustainability issues. They identify innovative thinking, promote networking, coordinate events, and facilitate the implementation of new projects and the spread of successful ones. It is a model that isn't exactly either top-down or bottom-up; it is a dynamic networked approach to mapping pathways to health and sustainability.

Also in the mix are companies in a position to organize consumer purchasing. Examples here include Carrotmob, Groupon, and LivingSocial.

Carrotmob arranges for businesses to compete based on how socially responsible they can be, and participating consumers reward the businesses that make the best offer. Their campaigns are the opposite of a boycott. They line up orderly mobs of consumers who want to use their dollars to help make socially responsible corporate practices more profitable.

Groupon and LivingSocial enlist competing local businesses to bid for a crowd of buyers that is willing to buy what the companies are willing to offer. The typical bid links a guaranteed low price to a guaranteed minimum number of buyers. The business with the winning bid then appears on the Groupon or Living Social websites as a daily deal. Users can track the website, Facebook, or Twitter for daily deal announcements. Users form a crowd of consumers that will send their cash into a chosen business using coupon codes or printed vouchers.

Groupon and LivingSocial arrange trades between price and sales volume. Unlike Carrotmob, they have yet to arrange many deals in terms that trade social and environmental responsibility for sales volume. It seems unlikely that doing so would cause companies to lose business. If anything, it should improve their ability to compete and grow. Interested users would simply look for the daily deals that, as part of the bargain, added value in the form of verifiable acts of corporate responsibility.

Corporate responsibility could mean local recycling, shifting inventory to include more free-trade items, donations of a share of profits to a cause, green-friendly initiatives, coalition building, or anything else the parties negotiate. Success would depend on connections with company insiders able to supply a realistic read on what is possible with the right kind of nudge on the right kind of issue. Opening new channels for consumers to express their moral materialism would almost effortlessly advance the cause of health and sustainability.

At *onebodymind.com*, we want to lend a hand to all people, circles, groups, and organizations willing to participate in the climb toward health and sustainability. We are in search of wisdom and new ideas on how to make personal and social wellness an emotionally engaging and enjoyable team effort.

If we remain flexible and open to the possibility that our parts can work together to make a healthier whole, if we believe in our capacity to heal and sustain our collective relationship to the world, we will provide service not only to Earth system science and the causes of human flourishing, but to a Maker as well. Faith and reason would become mutually reinforcing sources of idealistic inspiration and realistic hope that gives us the courage and confidence we need to support the functional integrity of the greater whole in which we have our being. If we are to succeed in realizing our highest social ideals as a species, we must rely on realistic appraisals of what will work to stimulate heroic habits at personal and social levels within our cultures.

The Romantic poet and philosopher Samuel Taylor Coleridge (1772–1834) observed that, "He [or she] is the best physician who is the most ingenious inspirer of hope." Coleridge assuredly was not talking about false hope but about hope that is deep, genuine, and abiding because it is firmly rooted in reality. Yet reality has a mystical, metaphysical side that encourages us to remain humble about what we can know about the mysterious source of our being.

A good planetary medicine doctor wouldn't think to approach a healing task without a desire to base hope on a realistic assessment of what's going on within the system as a whole—but the physician's task is also to confront the ambiguity that exists between what is "known" and what is "real." The robe of medicine drapes the physician in humility. Medicine is a tireless campaign to humbly wield an idealistic realism against illness and suffering in pursuit of the functional integrity that living systems need to maintain their health and sustainability.

The human bodymind acquired its energetic, molecular, cellular, metabolic, rational, and intuitive forms of wisdom over an arc of time that stretches back some 13.7 billion years to when the form was void. The bodymind of humanity is only beginning to develop the collective wisdom it needs to adapt and survive the perils of modernity. But it may do so quickly, in the span of a few generations, if swarms of professional-level amateurs, conscientious consumer-citizens, and virtuoso gamers bring their heroic habits to a quest that, along the way, must drive cultural institutions to use their power and influence in ways that support a healthier, more sustainable way of being in the world.

From the standpoint of a planetary medicine doctor, learned optimism gives us reasons to trust that with creativity, patience, and persistence, clinical reasoning can yield deeply hoped-for results despite seemingly insurmountable odds. By combining the zoom lens methodologies of the reductionist with the wide-angle models of the integrative scientist; by using an integrative clinical mind-set that is free to move from the evidence of controlled studies to the free-thinking wisdom of inductive logic, experience, intuition, and the thoughtfully staged empirical trial; by giving consumers seats on a panel of experts that for too long has relied on leaders in science, politics, and industry alone—we can solve many of the humanity's toughest problems.

If sound clinical reasoning can work for a case of intractable eczema, who says it can't work for a case of intractable anthropocentric anxiety? Both are just problems within living systems with solutions waiting to be found.

Reinhold Niebuhr (1892–1971), H. Richard Niebuhr's older brother, is credited with coining the first widely circulated version of what's now known as the Serenity Prayer. He was, and remains, widely admired for his theological, moral, and political insights, including the idea that humankind would always struggle to make the world a better place if left to its own authority.

He observed that groups condone immorality more than individuals because the moral responsibility for any harms caused get diffused within the group, making it easier to deflect accountability. He relied on this observation to partially explain the extreme lack of moral accountability within the Third Reich. He felt that it helped account for why human societies have a perfect track record for being imperfectible. If corporations are people, they are people with a built-in reason to avoid accountability for the harms they cause to others.

At the same time, we depend on social cooperation to achieve things that we cannot accomplish on our own. How are we to navigate between the rocks of our social weaknesses and our social needs?

Niebuhr argued that we should not trust ourselves, or our social institutions, to find a path that leads to human flourishing. Unable to self-correct misuses of power by groups, yet unable to act alone without the help of social institutions, Niebuhr argued

that we should defer to a third-party source for guidance. Here's
how he put it in his book *Moral Man and Immoral Society*:

> Nothing worth doing is completed in our lifetime; therefore
> we must be saved by Hope. Nothing true or beautiful makes
> complete sense in any immediate context of history; therefore
> we must be saved by Faith. Nothing we do, however virtuous,
> can be accomplished alone; therefore, we are saved by Love.

Hope, faith, and love must be our companions on the road
to health and sustainability, or we will not make it. In a universe
that insists at the very least on the *possibility* of God, we have
no license to be anything but humble about navigating life on
our own authority, especially when we are mastered by emotions
whose influences on our behavior we barely understand or control.

Few writers have captured the implications of unconscious
emotion in human judgment and choice better than David Brooks
has in *The Social Animal*. Brooks, a respected columnist and opinion leader by day, is a formidable moral and political philosopher
by night. *The Social Animal* heads my list of required reading for
people who want to understand why some relationships work and
others don't, and why the determinants of our social successes and
failures are often impossible to pin down, yet still decipherable in
terms of their main patterns.

A problem, *causal indeterminacy*, plagues our studies of the
human bodymind. Biology, psychology, and sociology blur into
each other creating what University of Virginia behavioral genet-
icist Eric Turkheimer calls *the gloomy prospect*—our seemingly
permanent inability to tease apart cause from effect concerning
human development and behavior.

Brooks does his best to make the forecast look less gloomy.
He slips well-chosen research insights into his descriptions of the

root dynamics of the relationship between a fictional husband and wife. At one point early on in the story, he presents a profoundly rich vignette showing the patience of a mother trying to help her disorganized son, Harold, with his homework. Her directive teaching style is an utter failure. Harold has a fit. Once the eruption settles down, "She instinctively pulled him in, and brought him a bit inside her own life." She told him a story about a road trip she took with some friends after college.

Stressed and disorganized Harold is now rapt with attention, learning new information that naturally matters to him, with his mother speaking to him as if he were her companion on a wondrous journey as opposed to a scatterbrained kid with an uncontrollable temper. The effect "was like a miracle." Harold gathered himself together and smoothly finished his homework. This parenting method has never been proven to conquer attention deficit problems in well-designed trials but its immediate applicability rings like a bell to parents in similar situations because there is common sense wisdom in it.

Brooks elaborates:

But of course it wasn't a miracle. If there is one thing developmental psychologists have learned over the years, it is that parents don't have to be brilliant psychologists to succeed. They don't have to be supremely gifted teachers. Most of the stuff parents do with flashcards and special drills and tutorials to hone their kids into perfect achievement machines don't have any effect at all. Instead, parents just have to be good enough. They have to provide their kids with stable and predictable rhythms. They need to be able to fall in tune with their kids' needs, combining warmth and discipline. They need to establish the secure emotional bonds that kids can fall

back upon in the face of stress. They need to be there to provide living examples of how to cope with the problems of the
world so that their children can develop unconscious models
in their heads.

Brooks then shares what various child psychologists have
determined about the quality of the attachments made between
parents and their children. Most children fall into one of three
main categories:

1. *Securely attached.* This pattern does not depend so much
   on parenting styles so much as attunement and an ability
   to mirror a child's shifting moods, providing comfort and
   support as needed. These children grow into adults who
   cope and handle stressful situations well. They tend to be
   open to meeting new people and forming affiliations.

2. *Avoidantly attached.* This pattern occurs more frequently
   when the parents are emotionally withdrawn or psycho-
   logically detached from their children's anxieties. These
   children can figure out how to care for themselves, but
   they end up preferring to go it alone rather than ask others for help and risk an attachment that could sting.

3. *Ambivalently attached.* This pattern correlates with parents who tune in and out. Warm one minute, cold the
   next, intrusive on one day, helpful the next. Such emotional disorganization creates intense approach-avoidance
   conflicts in kids. They want mom or dad to be a faithful
   companion, but they're afraid of getting hurt again. The
   rhythms of the home are not predictable. These children
   tend to be fearful, untrusting, and impulsive as adults.

Attachment patterns set the mold for future inclinations toward being socially cooperative. Securely attached children have long emotional leashes and will likely face the adventure of life head-on. Avoidantly attached children have short emotional leashes; they're anxious about venturing out too far, happiest on their own in the spot in the yard they know and trust. Ambivalently attached children struggle to find happiness. They'd rather avoid the outside world. When they do enter it, they often follow their impulses in ways that are inexplicable to other people. If our long-term health and sustainability depends on reaching new heights in social cooperation, job one is to support the formation of secure attachments between parents and children. It may well be our species' highest priority.

Brooks' work is a valuable source of insight into how the unconscious mind drives behavior and funds the formation of character and emotional self-control; it also clarifies how important proper emotional care of children is to the health and sustainability of life on our planet. For the planetary medicine doctor concerned about human flourishing and the sustainability of life in the Earth system, perhaps no issue matters more than the one that begins as a relationship between parents—or parental figures—and children.

If we can make our parent-child attachments secure, ethical character will become a stronger force in our cultures, and our lives will be made better because we became more willing to cooperate toward realizing shared ideals. The balance we seek in our social lives, and in our relationship to the world's other living systems, will be a product of the kind of children we raise. The kind of children we raise will be a product of how we master the controls of our own emotional development. We should want to feel securely attached to the Earth system the way our children want to be securely attached to us.

The most epic game of the twenty-first century is to turn a Balkanized game of thrones into a unified quest for health and sustainability. This is the game that will define the character of humanity for ages to come. Combatants will lose the game and destroy themselves in the process if they insist on making the game a usual and customary bout staged by politics among nations. Only cooperators can win the game. At present, there are not enough to go around. The first step is to recruit more cooperators to the quest.

The premise of the game is simple: figure out how we can live long and prosper together by finding healthy and sustainable solutions to the problems that stand in our way.

You misunderstand the premise of the game if you let problems sit on the back burner because science hasn't yet settled the matter to your satisfaction, or because political or religious solutions will drop out of the sky. Ignore the precautionary principle—the cardinal virtue of prudence—and the law of unintended consequences could take you and your species out. Denial and delay of valid claims adds drag when thrust is needed in our efforts to find integrative solutions to complex problems. Will an action or a strategy add or detract to some aspect of functional integrity within the whole? This is the key question we must hold in our minds as we prepare to set out on our quest.

You misunderstand the premise of the game if you think wellness innovators can only sit by and watch as our cash burning chronic disease paradigm charbroils America's hopes for a prosperous future. You misunderstand the premise of the game if you underestimate what an empowered consumer force can do to change reform-resistant institutions. By misunderstanding the premise of the game, you add to the risk that our species won't achieve the social transformation needed to get us to the next level. Letting your team down needs to mean letting billions of fellow human beings down, not too mention the astoundingly complex and beautiful living systems upon which our species depends. We must hold courage in our hearts as we prepare to set out on our quest.

Where else, then, beyond faith, reason, and ethics shall we turn for ideas about how to get straight with the premise of the world's most epic game, and with mapping out a strategy that can muster the heroic habits we'll need to win functional integrity, health, and sustainability?

We can turn to the wisdom of the human bodymind, where we find natural intelligence in action, distilled over the eons, the wisdom of ancient molecular pathways that produced the living systems that evolved into us. Even though we may not feel so genetically related, we can find common ground in the ninety-nine percent of the human genome that all people share, just as we find that ninety-nine percent of all people share a desire to be healthy and well.

In the wisdom of the human bodymind, we will find examples of integrated systems working together as a team to serve the health of a greater whole; we will find patterns and processes of interdependence worth emulating at the level of our cultural systems and social institutions.

The metabolic wisdom of your bodymind is where you will find the most powerful medicine in the world. By exploring and understanding what's going on within you, you will learn important lessons about how to value health not just for yourself, but also at other levels within the living systems that surround you.

A new vision for health and healing is emerging that applies to all living systems at once. This vision summons deep and difficult questions about what health is and how we should go about creating, maintaining, and restoring it. Then where better to turn for answers to such questions than to our system of health care? That's what a health care system is for, right, to handle our deepest concerns about health?

Excuse me. I have to throw up.

America's health care system, as great as it is in so many ways, still falls nauseatingly short of its potential to be a fully realized force for healing. It waits until disease is already firmly established before it jumps to the rescue with drugs, procedures, and other measures so costly that they are bankrupting families and dragging down businesses and governments. In an effort to control costs physicians are being forced into a corner where they use one arm to administer to patients and the other to swordfight with insurance companies. So many physicians and patients are feeling abused by a care process that is ostensibly designed to promote healing.

Doctors can see the trenches being dug for them. The health care sector is morphing into a battlefield dominated by corporate superpowers. Pesky doctors have had their day in the sun. They can now swear fealty to the axis of insurers that already controls cash flow and working conditions for most members of the medical profession, or they can fend for themselves. Patients, as always, are helpless onlookers relegated to the sidelines, about to become collateral damage yet again, their fates determined not by themselves but by cost-shifting behemoths with their own agendas.

The next book in this series, *Value Health*, explores the root dynamics of illness that prevail in our formidably disjointed health system, seeking to explain why the American health care sector has become a busy but hollow realm of gleaming castles where disruptive forms of divergent thinking go to die.

Bibliography

◇◇◇◇◇◇◇◇◇◇◇◇◇◇◇◇◇◇◇◇◇◇◇◇◇◇◇◇◇◇◇◇◇◇◇◇

Armstrong, John. 2010. *Your Church Is Too Small.* Zondervan: Grand Rapids, MI.

Baker, Sidney MacDonald. 2003. *Detoxification and Healing.* 2nd ed. McGraw-Hill: New York.

Bell, Rob. 2011. *Love Wins: A Book About Heaven, Hell, and the Fate of Every Person Who Ever Lived.* HarperCollins: New York.

Bland, Jeffrey. 1999. *Genetic Nutritioneering.* Keats: Lincolnwood, IL.

Bourke, Andrew F. G. 2011. *The Principles of Social Evolution.* Oxford University Press: New York.

Brafman, Ori, and Rod A. Beckstrom. 2010. *The Starfish and the Spider: The Unstoppable Power of Leaderless Organizations.* Penguin: New York.

Brooks, David. 2011. *The Social Animal: The Hidden Sources of Love, Character, and Achievement.* Random House: New York.

Carr, Nicholas. 2010. *The Shallows: What the Internet Is Doing to Our Brains.* W. W. Norton: New York.

Cervantes. [1605] 2003. *Don Quixote.* Penguin Classics: New York.

Chivian, Eric, and Aaron Bernstein, eds. 2008. *Sustaining Life: How Human Health Depends on Biodoversity.* Oxford University Press: New York.

Christensen, Clayton, Jerome Grossman, and Jason Hwang. 2008. *The Innovator's Prescription.* McGraw-Hill: New York.

Christian, David. 2005. *Maps of Time: An Introduction to Big History.* University of California Press: Berkeley.

Collier, Paul. 2010. *The Plundered Planet: Why We Must—and How We Can—Manage Nature for Global Prosperity.* Oxford University Press: New York.

Collins, Francis. 2006. *The Language of God: A Scientist Presents Evidence for Belief.* Free Press: New York.

Collins, Francis. 2010. *Belief: Readings on the Reason for Faith.* Harper Collins: New York

Conway Morris, Simon. 2008. Evolution and Convergence: Some Wider Considerations. In *The Deep Structure of Biology: Is Convergence Sufficiently Ubiquitous to Give a Directional Signal?* edited by Simon Conway Morris. Templeton Foundation Press: West Conshohocken, PA.

Crouch, Andy. 2008. *Culture Making: Recovering Our Creative Calling.* Intervarsity Press: Downer's Grove, IL.

Davison Hunter, James. 2010. *To Change the World: The Irony, Tragedy, and Possibility of Christianity in the Late Modern World.* Oxford University Press: New York.

Dawkins, Richard. 1976. *The Selfish Gene*. Oxford University Press: New York.

Dennett, Daniel. 2003. *Freedom Evolves*. Penguin: New York.

Florida, Richard. 2010. *The Great Reset*. HarperCollins: New York.

Freedman, David H. 2010. Lies, Damned Lies, and Medical Science. *The Atlantic Monthly*, November.

Friedman, Thomas. 2010. Global Weirding Is Here. *New York Times*, February 17.

Gawande, Atul. 2002. *Complications: A Surgeon's Notes on an Imperfect Science*. Picador: New York.

Gediman, Dan, and John Gregory. 2010. *Edward R. Murrow's This I Believe*. This I Believe, http://thisibelieve.org.

Gladwell, Malcolm. 2008. *Outliers: The Story of Success*. Little Brown: New York.

Gustafson, James M. 1981. *Ethics from a Theocentric Perspective*. Volume 1. University of Chicago Press: Chicago.

Gustafson, James M. 1984. *Ethics from a Theocentric Perspective*. Volume 2. University of Chicago Press: Chicago.

Hamilton, W. D. 1996. *Narrow Roads of Gene Land*. Volumes 1 and 2. Oxford University Press: New York.

Haught, John F. 2008. Purpose in Nature: On the Possibility of a Theology of Evolution. In *The Deep Structure of Biology: Is Convergence Sufficiently Ubiquitous to Give a Directional Signal?* Simon Conway Morris, ed. Templeton Foundation Press: West Conshohocken, PA.

Hayes, T. B., V. R. Beasley, S. de Solla, T. Iguchi, et al. 2011. Demasculinization and Feminization of Male Gonads by

Atrazine: Consistent Effects across Vertebrate Classes. *Journal of Steroid Biochemistry and Molecular Biology*. Online publication date March 22.

Hayes, T. B., K. Haston, M. Tsui, A. Hoang, et al. 2003. Atrazine-induced Hermaphrodism at 0.1 ppb in American Leopard Frogs (*Rana pipiens*): Laboratory and Field Evidence. *Environmental Health Perspectives*. 111:568–575.

Hill, Austin Bradford. 1965. Environment and disease: association or causation? *Proceedings of the Royal Society of Medicine*. 58(5) May:295-300.

Hume, David. 1751. *An Enquiry Concerning the Principles of Morals*. Neeland Media, Lawrence, KS. Amazon.com Kindle edition.

Ioannidis, John P. A. 2005. Why Most Published Research Findings Are False. *Public Library of Science* 2(8):e124.

Kabat-Zinn, Jon, Davidson, Richard J., and Houshmand, Zara. 2011. *The Mind's Own Physician: A Scientific Dialogue with the Dalai Lama on the Healing Power of Meditation*. New Harbinger Publications: Oakland, CA.

Kant, Immanuel. [1792] 1960. *Religion within the Limits of Reason Alone*. Translated by Theodore M. Green and Hoyt H. Hudson. Harper Torchbooks: New York.

Kolbert, Elizabeth. 2011. Storms Brewing. *The New Yorker*, June 13 and 20.

Lehrer, Jonah. 2010. The Truth Wears Off: Is There Something Wrong with Scientific Method? *The New Yorker*, December 13, 52–57.

Lloyd, Seth. 2006. *Programming the Universe: A Quantum Computer Scientist Takes On the Cosmos*. Alfred P. Knopf: New York.

McGonigal, Jane. 2011. *Reality Is Broken: Why Games Make Us Better and How They Can Change the World.* Penguin Press HC: New York.

Mitchell, Melanie. 2009. *Complexity: A Guided Tour.* Oxford University Press: New York.

Niebuhr, Reinhold. 1932. *Moral Man and Immoral Society: A Study in Ethics and Politics.* Charles Scribner and Sons: New York.

Niebuhr, Richard. 1963. *The Responsible Self.* Harper and Row: New York.

Pagels, Heinz. 1989. *The Dreams of Reason.* Bantam: New York.

Pew Research Center poll. 2009. *Scientists and Belief.* The Pew Forum on Religion and Public Life.

Pink, Daniel. 2006. *A Whole New Mind: Why Right-Brainers Will Rule the Future.* Penguin: New York.

Pope, Stephen J. 2007. *Human Evolution and Christian Ethics.* Cambridge University Press: New York.

Reeder, A. L., M. O. Ruiz, A. Pessier, L. E. Brown, et al. 2005. Intersexuality and the Cricket Frog Decline: Historic and Geographical Trends. *Environmental Health Perspectives* 113(3):261–265.

Reid, W. V., D. Chen, L. Goldfard, et al. Earth System Science for Global Sustainability: Grand Challenges. *Science,* November 12, 2010, 916–917.

Rescher, Nicholas. 2002. An Idealistic Realism: Presuppositional Realism and Justificatory Idealism. In *The Blackwell Guide to Metaphysics.* Richard M. Gale, ed. Blackwell: London.

Ridley, Matt. 2010. *The Rational Optimist: How Prosperity Evolves.* HarperCollins: New York.

Royal Society. 2011. *Knowledge, Networks, and Nations: Global Scientific Collaboration in the 21st Century.* RS policy document 03/11.

Santayana, George. [1905] 1980. *The Life of Reason.* Dover Publications: New York.

Schweitzer, Albert. 2002. *Reverence for Life.* Marvin Meyer and Kurt Begel, eds. Syracuse University Press: Syracuse, New York.

Shirky, Clay. 2010. *Cognitive Surplus: Creativity and Generosity in a Connected Age.* Penguin: New York.

Smith, John Maynard, and Erös Szathmány. 1995. *The Major Transitions in Evolution.* Oxford University Press: New York.

Smith, John Maynard, and Erös Szathmány. 1999. *The Origins of Life.* Oxford University Press: New York.

Teilhard de Chardin, Pierre. 1999. *The Human Phenomenon.* Translated by Sarah Appleton-Weber. Sussex Academic Press: Portland.

Tillich, Paul. 1964. *The Courage To Be.* Yale University Press: New York.

Tzu, Lao. 1996. *The Tao Te Ching.* Translated by Brian Brown Walker. St. Martin's Griffin: New York.

Van De Walle, J., et al. 2010. Deoxynivalenol Affects In Vitro Epithelial Barrier Integrity through Inhibition of Protein Synthesis. *Toxicology and Applied Pharmacology* 245:291–298.

Playlist

◇◇◇◇◇◇◇◇◇◇◇◇◇◇◇◇◇◇◇◇◇◇◇◇◇◇◇◇◇◇◇◇◇◇◇

Evil

3:35

Written and performed by Stevie Wonder

From the album *Music of My Mind*

©1972 Universal/Motown Records Group

Wise Up

3:21

Written and performed by Aimee Mann

From the album *Magnolia: Music from the Motion Picture*

©1999 Reprise

The Sound of Muzak

4:59

Written and performed by Porcupine Tree

From the album *In Absentia*

©2002 Lava Records

You Dance

3:57

Written and performed by East Mountain South

From the album *East Mountain South*

©2003 Dreamworks

Peace Be Upon Us

4:22

Written and performed by Sheryl Crow

From the album *Detours*

©2008 A&M

About the Author

◇◇◇◇◇◇◇◇◇◇◇◇◇◇◇◇◇◇◇◇◇◇◇◇◇◇◇◇◇◇◇◇◇◇◇◇

Keith Berndtson, MD, practices integrative medicine in Park Ridge, Illinois. In 1996, after ten years in family medicine and corporate health, he chose a road less traveled. On this road he came to realize the wisdom and value of the integrative and functional medicine traditions. He uses this experience to explore the wider implications of a clinical systems biology approach to wellness.

His medical practice, Park Ridge MultiMed, uses functional medicine principles to evaluate and treat patients with medically unexplained and non-responsive forms of chronic illness.

Berndtson founded *onebodymind.com* to supply innovative online tools for people interested in a deeper, more effective approach to health education, self-care support, and the stewardship of living systems. The website is also ground zero for a social network that will help prepare the way for the modern quest for health and sustainability.

Cover/Permissions/Figures

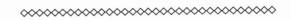

Cover:

CreateSpace

Permissions:

Wallace Stegner interview—This I Believe, Inc.

Table:

Adapted from the 2009 Pew Research Center poll, *Scientists and Belief*.

Figure:

Concept by Keith Berndtson, MD; diagram by Kristin Wienandt.

Made in the USA
San Bernardino, CA
14 December 2013